It is not stress that kills us,

it is our reaction to it.

Hans Seyle

For my lovely husband

Thanks for... everything in the world;

but most of all, for self belief and peace.

I love you more than you will ever know

Introduction

Stress is pandemic in our society. Doctors agree it plays a massive part in serious and chronic disease in our culture. Heart disease, type 2 diabetes and strokes are all very real and present dangers for people suffering from stress. Stress is an incredibly dangerous thing.

People now accept aromatherapists can alleviate stress and will happily trundle along for an aromatherapy massage for half an hour to relax. Little do they know; a person skilled in essential oils is capable of so much more.

Oils can clear toxicity, they can relax the mind and body and they can balance the organs and glands which are pumping these lethal poisons around the body.

If you like, you can call this book *The Off Switch*.

But I think this work is the **On**-*Switch*....for the turbo boost your business needs.

I'll teach you the skills to go deeper and deeper into stress related problems and how to peel back the layers of their disease. I'll share with you oils which detoxify the system of fertilisers and petrochemicals and explain why these will transform how you treat your patients.

The book reveals how to nourish their system back to health and even shares vitamins therapy, acupressure points and dietary strategies to get your patient well. I'll show you why you should legitimately be seeing your clients at least four times more often than you have been doing (making you at least four times more money than you do now!) and I'll explain why simply relaxing them will not make them better.

If you are looking for a book on relaxation, you need to search again. That's not what I do. If you are looking for a way to build on your existing knowledge and learn cold, hard, clinical healing, then congratulations, I'm your gal.

Here's what you should already know

- Essential oils affect the emotions
- They can be used by inhaling them or by absorbance through the skin
- They affect changes in the mind but can also ones in the physical body too
- They can alter hormonal balances
- They can heal a person's well being
- Everyone has subtle bodies of an aura and chakras too. These connect the spirit to the physical body.
- But most of all...many essential oils smell utterly delicious.

Here's what should *also* know.

If there is one single point in the list which is new...then you need this book. It will transform the potential of your business to treat the largest client field available.

- Essential oils work on the mind, the body and the spirit. If any one of these is dis-eased then symptoms will show in the patient's physical body

- Stress is the number one factor in type 2 diabetes, heart disease, high blood pressure and strokes because it sends toxicity to the liver and adrenal glands which causes other related functions such as the pituitary, kidneys and pancreas to falter. If you know which essential oils to use you can detoxify the system to alleviate these effects.

- Some traumas get stuck in the brain processing, as well as the bodily tissues, making it impossible for the patient to heal. It is possible to use essential oils to mimic one of psychiatry's most revolutionary practices to move PTSD patients out of their shell and then start healing.

- The aura and chakras give indicators of where this disease could emanate from and translate illness to the physical body. Essential oils eradicate possible effects by dealing with the emotional and spiritual distress before it reaches physical manifestation.

- Healing cannot be fully successful unless a patient's spine is straight. Any misalignments will potentially cause dis-ease to continue.

- Stress starves vitamins from the body, which is usually under-nourished anyway because of poor diet or from our 21st century substandard foods. Any disturbance of minerals in the body causes a ricochet of imbalance through the system. By understanding which minerals may be misfiring, we can nourish a person back to health.

- Most western bodies are already fighting a losing battle because of toxaemia from an onslaught of static, heavy metals and petrochemicals, pharmaceuticals, light pollution and noise. This book tells you how to detoxify the system of all of these to strengthen your patients' systems for further onslaughts of stress.

- Whilst you can alleviate the effects of stress, the actual pressures of life never actually go away. Understand the strategies for referral or treatment to make your patient more resilient to the rigours of everyday life.

- Most people are stressed because of huge demands on them from the economy, from the media and from familial expectations. Many though are unhappy since they actually have forgotten how to be joyful, or perhaps they never even knew.

- The vast percentage of people are so busy being who they think they should be they forget just how it feels being themselves, doing what comes naturally to them and using their innate skills.

There is very little healing knowledge in this book which the Jill Bruce School of Aromatherapy did not teach back in '93. In fact, a great deal comes straight from my Advanced Aromatherapy lesson notes. The thing is though: the public's perception of the art has changed. They *know* what aromatherapy is now...especially in terms of stress. The problem is therapists are still not equipped to deal with either the public's or the doctors' new found acceptances of it.

Aromatherapy is no longer fringe science. It has clinical trials backing it up, funding in hospitals, and when hospices and special schools run out of ideas, they turn to us.

What's more, the internet, marketing's greatest ally could potentially be aromatherapy's hugest threat. Much of the information out there is rehashed rubbish of the same old information. Many of Amazon's books are written by people who have never picked up a bottle of oil let alone treated someone who was sick. Consequently although I can give you real evidence that people want to know more about what you do, they go away feeling frankly despondent about what they read. They seek other therapies to sort out their problems.

This is why to me, this book is vital. Without it, I fear the healing art which I believe vehemently in, will be lost again in the mire.

So here's what I can offer you.

- The knowledge to fill the healing gaps which improve your patient results exponentially.
- The wisdom of which oils to use.
- I'll introduce you to professionals who can help you in your journey to make your patient's well.
- Best of all you will see your business achieve the potential you always knew it could, but sadly have been watching in frustration and bewilderment as somehow it just *wouldn't*.

Right here, right now this is about to change.

Welcome to the ***Professional Stress Solution***.

Table of Contents

Chapter 1 The Physiology of Stress

I think everyone now understands how dangerous stress is to their health. We all know someone who is worrying themselves into a heart attack or is about to give themselves an ulcer. But how does that happen and how on earth can we stop it happening to us? In the *Mind Body Spirit of Clinical Aromatherapy,* we looked at how the bodymind runs through the body, and how emotions can affect heath.

Here, we are going to look at the physiological processes which are affected by stress, focusing on the brain itself. There are very few occasions where I point out the overlap between the two, mainly because it will become inordinately confusing, but throughout this book always keep in your mind that the brain (as an organ) affects the body, but also that the mind and body are, most certainly, one and the same.

What is stress?

The term stress was first coined in the 1930s by Hans Seyle. Prior to this it had been an engineering term pertaining to how well a substance could cope with pressure.

Now in *humans* it's a quite a hard term to define I suppose, because *your* stress will be very different to *mine*. My eldest son is the most chilled out person on the planet, he breezes his uni work with ease. Laid back doesn't even come close to describing his manner....until the student finance forms come.

He panics so much he becomes impossible to live with. It is entirely out of character, so I wanted to understand why.

"Because something always goes wrong, mum."

I'd like to say he was wrong but let's just say the online form and I have a *difficult* history. I will admit there have been glitches and screw ups and far more four letter words than I would care to own up to my dad about, but not enough to warrant the knee trembling horror student finance frankly gives *both* of us now.

Here's the thing. It has become *far bigger* in both of our minds.

And whilst stress isn't a medical diagnosis, it sure **is** a recognised condition.

So what sorts of things make it worse?

Timescales definitely do; too much to do, too little time....Recognise that one?

Other people's expectations...whether that is our boss with new targets, our husband who forgets there are other things in life outside of ordering his paper, or wives who refuse to stop spending. These are blazing generalisations but you get the picture.

So, to take it a bit further then: could we assume we become stressed because things feel out of our control?

This could also be true. This hypothesis is backed up by workplace studies which show that workers on the bottom rung of the ladder experience the most chronic forms of stress because they feel they are unable to exert any degree of control on their surroundings.

Do you want to know what the worst protagonist of my stress is? *Oh yes!* I should point out that The Secret Healer is not even close to a serene transcendental-levitating-yogic-flying-peaceful-being...I can out-stress the best of them. The only difference between me and the person becoming ill through stress is that I have discovered the off switch.

So, for a moment, let's just think about what causes our own stress. What's my worst stressor?

Me.

I set myself unrealistic workloads. I want my output to be bigger, better and brighter than anyone else's. No-one truly could live up to expectations I impose on myself.

How many of you can relate to that?

Thankfully I have a great pool of people around me who just laugh in my face when I do it, and then they point out that I, perhaps, really need to get a grip.

Stress and health

Ok. So we understand the concept of stress, but how does that translate into the poor health a patient experiences?

At this point I am going to add in a disclaimer because in some ways these notes about physiology make sweeping generalisations about health, because not everyone reacts to health in the same way. I could write a book full of "coulda, woulda, shoulda lead to this that and the other", but it makes a terribly laborious read.

Richard Bryant at the University of New South Wales has identified why some of us react in a worse way to stress than others. It seems certain people are born with a shorter version of the serotonin transport gene. These people are at higher risk of depression and potentially will also take longer to heal.

My point being, every person is different; however the principle processes of the physiology of stress are not. Follow the guidelines and you won't go far wrong.

We also need to make the distinction between **acute stress** which will be a one off traumatic event (or the anticipation or expectation of one- like moving house, for instance) and

chronic stress. If a person undergoes even minimal stress for a long and protracted period it can turn into chronic stress. These are the patients you will see most and this is the focus of this book.

So for the effects of short term or acute stress we could be referring to the suddenly vital run to the toilet before a driving test, but longer term expectations of chronic stress can be heart attack or stroke.

Other symptoms of stress are myriad.

Are you ready for this?

According to the American Institute of Stress, symptoms you may need to watch out for are:

- *Frequent headaches, jaw clenching or pain*
- *Gritting, grinding teeth*
- *Stuttering or stammering*
- *Tremors, trembling of lips, hands*
- *Neck ache, back pain, muscle spasms*
- *Light headedness, faintness, dizziness*
- *Ringing, buzzing or "popping sounds"*
- *Frequent blushing, sweating*
- *Cold or sweaty hands, feet*
- *Dry mouth, problems swallowing*
- *Frequent colds, infections, herpes sores*

- *Rashes, itching, hives, "goose bumps"*
- *Unexplained or frequent "allergy" attacks*
- *Heartburn, stomach pain, nausea*
- *Excess belching, flatulence*
- *Constipation, diarrhea, loss of control*
- *Difficulty breathing, frequent sighing*
- *Sudden attacks of life threatening panic*
- *Chest pain, palpitations, rapid pulse*
- *Frequent urination*
- *Diminished sexual desire or performance*
- *Excess anxiety, worry, guilt, nervousness*
- *Increased anger, frustration, hostility*
- *Depression, frequent or wild mood swings*
- *Increased or decreased appetite*
- *Insomnia, nightmares, disturbing dreams*
- *Difficulty concentrating, racing thoughts*
- *Trouble learning new information*
- *Forgetfulness, disorganization, confusion*
- *Difficulty in making decisions*
- *Feeling overloaded or overwhelmed*
- *Frequent crying spells or suicidal thoughts*
- *Feelings of loneliness or worthlessness*
- *Little interest in appearance, punctuality*
- *Nervous habits, fidgeting, feet tapping*
- *Increased frustration, irritability, edginess*

- *Overreaction to petty annoyances*
- *Increased number of minor accidents*
- *Obsessive or compulsive behaviour*
- *Reduced work efficiency or productivity*
- *Lies or excuses to cover up poor work*
- *Rapid or mumbled speech*
- *Excessive defensiveness or suspiciousness*
- *Problems in communication, sharing*
- *Social withdrawal and isolation*
- *Constant tiredness, weakness, fatigue*
- *Frequent use of over-the-counter drugs*
- *Weight gain or loss without diet*
- *Increased smoking, alcohol or drug use*
- *Excessive gambling or impulse buying*

Phew! What a list. Now as I go down it some have obvious protagonists, others not so much. Why, for instance, might sexuality be reduced or belching be increased just because a patient feels stressed? To understand this we need to explore the physiology of stress.

The Physiology of stress

It seems sensible to write here: in some ways, it is problematic for me not to know the training benchmark of each of my readers. In that case then, those who read repetitions of their learning, please excuse me, and for those beginners I hope that

I do not go too fast! It is important we cover this fully as it will help you to understand how each part of the healing works.

I'll start by describing it fully in jargon and then I'll break it down into more simple terms. Don't worry if you don't get it immediately, because after the initial physiology it becomes far easier to understand.

The initial stress response is originally processed in the part of the brain called the **hippocampus**, which registers the existence of a potential danger and then passes it on to the *amygdala*. This interprets the <u>stress in terms of images and sounds</u> and then translates them to the **hypothalamus.** Meanwhile though, the vmPFC (**Ventromedial prefrontal cortex**), the centre of rational thought, aims to calm the amygdala by putting the imminent danger into some context.

When the hypothalamus receives danger signals, it then communicates these to the sympathetic nervous system. This, then, triggers the **Fight and Flight Response**; it does this by transmitting synapses along the autonomic nerves to the **adrenals**. All of this happens so quickly that a person might jump out the way of an oncoming car before they have even realised they have seen it coming.

The adrenals then pump the hormone *epinephrine* into the blood increasing, heart rate. As the epinephrine levels subside, the hypothalamus then activates what is called the HPA axis

(**H**ypothalamus, **P**ituitary, **A**drenals), which involves the hypothalamus triggering CRF (Corticotrophin Releasing Factor) to be released from the pituitary and then ACTH (adrenocorticotrophic hormone) from the adrenals. From this, the parasympathetic system then applies the brakes for the system to slow down.

Confused? You should be. Let's look at the glands and organs in turn. I find it helps to put them in reverse.

Let me first introduce you to a set of glands called:

The adrenals

These sit on top of each of your kidneys. They are part of a set of glands we call the endocrine system. Together the endocrines control the hormones in your body. We'll meet some of the others from the set later on.

The adrenals secrete many hormones, but the two we are most concerned with here are epinephrine (which is better known by the name adrenaline) and cortisol.

Adrenaline, I am sure most of you have heard of. In its most extreme case it's that rush you feel as the bungee rope pings back up, or the moment your parachute successfully opens. On a more mundane level, it's the feeling you get when you are running late for work....again.

We call the way your adrenals function, the Fight and Flight Syndrome, and really it is easiest to understand if we refer it back to the very beginnings of Man.

An ancient adrenal tale

Imagine our Neanderthal hero sitting in his cave and his pretty Neanderthal wife keeps on having a dig.

"When are you going to catch us something decent to eat? Neanderthal Nora down the rock got Mammoth yesterday, and what have we got again...barbecued rat! I bet she doesn't have to do her washing up in the same pot as she washes her clothes in. No-o-o, because Neanderthal Norman bought *her* a new pot last week..."

And so it continues until our Neanderthal Nigel can't take the ear bending any more. He takes up his spear and heads off into the wilderness.

Hours he treks, until eventually he hears a strange rumbling behind him. He turns and watching him is a sabre tooth tiger. A sabre tooth! That should keep the whining wife quiet for a few days!

Adrenaline kicks in.

His heart rate elevates, his pulse quickens and his breathing comes shallower. Strengthened by the rush of blood and extra oxygen supply, his muscles are far stronger than they would normally be. His legs run much faster and he leaps up the tree out of the predator's way, decidedly niftier than he would normally manage. An impressive sight he is too, all his bodily hair puffed up in display. His senses are sharpened and almost without thinking, he launches his spear and lances the sabre tooth smack between the eyes.

Dinner.

Which would be great; but now he has to get the wretched thing home. He looks at his watch....how long until someone invents a fork lift? He could really do with one now. In fact, he bets Neanderthal *Norman* has already got one for Nora!

It's heavy. It's cumbersome and he should be tired. But he's not. The adrenaline is still surging through his veins as he gets more and more enraged by his wife's obsession with Norman and how this should set the balance straight. He'd show her. Huh! Flamin' Mammoth! *So* last week!

The internal rant continues until he finds himself at the cave entrance. Dumping the tiger delicacy in the door way, he collapses in the corner exhausted. Not too bad though, he muses, he knows that look in Nagging Nancy's eye. Primitive our hero may be, but he knows a promise when he sees one.

Even the time it takes for the big cat to roast doesn't seem to bother her and Nigel can now relax. Dozing by the fire, he calms. Yep, life is pretty good, all things considered.

Present day pressure

The first thing to note is the obvious physical differences. Adrenaline still reacts in the same way. When we are excited (or cold) it still tries to puff up our body hair to protect us, but now the hair is gone. The astute among you will recognise that goose bumps still remain.

In every way, our bodies react in the same way as Nigel's did...except for one. We now have lives where it is impossible to kick out in front of the fire and let the hormones subside after exertion. No sooner has one stress gone, then we subject ourselves to the next bit again. And again. And again.

With no way to sustain or recharge them the adrenals eventually start to wane. They need to take their power from other places to cope.

There is also another hormone which, in effect, is the bodies back up plan to exhausted adrenaline levels and this is Norepinephrine. Again, it comes from the adrenals and also from the brain. Its job is arousal. The upside of this hormone is being alert and focused on the danger at hand. The downside, in simplistic terms, of having this in your blood is....little or no sleep.

So then let's think about:

Cortisol

Prepare to feel depressed and then to feel the penny drop about what your patients are experiencing starts to fall into place.

Cortisol's job is a survival tool. It makes sure if the body is threatened it can supply it with all the resources it needs to sustain itself.

The functions affected by cortisol levels are:

- Blood sugar (glucose) levels
- Fat, protein and carbohydrate metabolism to maintain blood glucose (gluconeogenesis)
- Immune responses
- Anti-inflammatory actions
- Blood pressure
- Heart and blood vessel tone and contraction
- Central nervous system activation

You can see how this, long term secretion of this hormone (with no off switch) might lead to exhausted immunity, diabetes or even a stroke.

The natural cycle of cortisol

For most people (I think 77%) there is a natural flow of cortisol through the day. We call this the CAR or Cortisol Awakening Response. That is, we rise in the morning, then 30-40 minutes later there is a spike of cortisol which gradually subsides throughout the day and is very low in the evening. Scientists suggest this to help us naturally have flow which will manage us through the day.

However stress causes anomalies, but stress is not the only thing. From a personal point of view, you may possibly recall my son and his hatred of Student Finance? He has Asperger's Syndrome. In 2009, The University of Bath established that [boys with] Aspergers's did not have the same cortisol cycle. They do not have a spike at all. This might explain why they need routine so much because they are not equipped with the mechanism to manage stress. Interestingly too, most Asperger's look far younger than their age and some hypothesize this maybe because they do not have cortisol wear and tear to age them. (I put "boys with" in [] because so far the assumption has only been tested on boys. Since the number of boys with the syndrome far outstrips the number of girls, perhaps this line will never be followed up).

"Another anomaly is found in babies. Scientists had originally thought that cortisol production established at about a year old, we now know this is not the case and that children are far older.

In a trial mothers were asked to take saliva swabs, to test cortisol levels four times daily: on awakening, then 30 minutes later and then again after their first nap and finally 30 minutes later.

The results were shocking. Rather than having a circadian rhythm as the adults had had, each baby's cortisol levels mimicked that of the mother's on every single test.

Now the connotations of this, in my mind, are massive. Clearly a stressed mother (or, I should probably say primary care giver) affects the cortisol levels and so thus, their child. Doctors agree that a child will have a greater chance of developing asthma or type 2 diabetes if they have had a stressful childhood. Could this be the reason why? I shall watch the labs with interest and wait.

I also think it is valuable to add here that more than half of patients with a condition called Cushing's Disease (a condition which presents many symptoms resulting from too much cortisol in the body) suffer from depression.

Even more interesting to those of you who, perhaps, treat any chronic conditions, is this. Prescribed anti inflammatory corticosteroids / hydrocortisone (the synthetic forms of cortisol) are known to be associated with the side effects of mild mood disorders. I investigate this in more detail in my book on eczema.

We know then, that acute stress is adaptive, your body can quickly recover from the effects. The long term effects of cortisol in the body through chronic stress however, can have deleterious effects on both behaviour and on health.

The amygdala

This is located in the brain. Like most organs and glands of the body, it is made up of two parts, the amygdalae. Their name comes from the ancient Greek which describes their shape: like an almond. They are located in the frontal lobe very close to the hippocampus.

The amygdala is vital to the way we feel certain emotions, in particular fear. It is also important for our ability to perceive emotions in others. In studies of patients who have experienced only injury to the amygdala (through strokes usually) they were able to identify every emotion behind photographs of facial expressions except for those of fear.

Now whilst regulating emotional responses and hormonal fluctuations associated with fear is certainly its primary response, we can say it is actually aligned to survival. Triggers for it include recognition of the presence of food, the proximity of a sexual partner; it warns of rivals and also activates when our children or loved ones are in distress.

Other functions of the amygdala are:

- Memory
- Decision making
- Emotional reactions

- Arousal

Studies by Harvard University have shown that the amygdala is not only *activated* by stress, but also undergoes semi-permanent changes if it is exposed to chronic stress.

In 2006 Paul Ardafio and Kwang Soo Kim published their preliminary findings of how cortisol affected two different groups of rats. Both groups were given doses of cortisol in their drinking water, one for just a day, the other group for two weeks.

The second group began to show semi permanent fear symptoms, being more reluctant to come out of their darkened shelter and explore their surroundings. This forms the basis of their ongoing search to create psychiatric drug which will treat the source of depression and stress, rather than its peripheral related diseases.

If you do any work with PTSD patients, you may be aware of Eye Movement Desensitizing and Re-programming (EMDR), which is a series of exercises done by a psychiatrist whilst the patient moves his eyes, up, down and across. Experiencing the memory during this movement helps to reprogram the fear response from the amygdala by bringing it forward and desensitizing the memory.

You may recall that the amygdala translates terror into images and sounds, which is exactly the horror of PTSD, this perpetual video play of their memories which will never cease. Most people will associate this with war, but you will also see it happen with people who come out of domestic violence situations as well as other very distressing events. The important clue here is that it is POST- traumatic.

The secondary horror of these memories usually happens some months after the event has passed. Scientists suggest this is due to the fact that the amygdala processes memories but does not store them long term and so there is a problem in the movement of the memories into the brains storage facility. Of all therapies for PTSD, EMDR proves to be the most successful.

vmPFC

We also know that *rational thought* is processed by the **prefrontal cortex**. Imagine for a moment you are in a zoo and a tiger comes and snarls at the bars. The amygdala shouts "Help its going to eat me" but the vmPFC tells you "wait a minute, you're in a zoo. There are bars to protect you and it's already had its lunch." It tries to keep the amygdala in check.

But, after weeks/months or years of being over ridden, the vmPFC kind of decides to go to sleep. In his book "The Feeling Of What Happens" Antonio Damasio investigates the relationship between abnormal activity of vmPFC and depression. We know that people who suffer from depression often experience low levels of activity in this area of the brain.

The VMPFC works in continuous flux sending messages back and forth to the amygdala. A person who shows problems with this area of their brain becomes unable to make rational long term decisions and moral judgments. They are also unable to regulate negative metal states but perhaps more problematically, **they also find it impossible to regulate cortisol.**

The hippocampus

Whilst cortisol stimulates the amygdala to grow new neurones, it actually stops neurones being added to the hippocampus. This means the hippocampus actually shrinks in size. As it decreases in power we find it harder to learn new things. Brain activity shifts from this area of the brain, over to where our emotions are processing worry. Consequently worries get bigger, bigger and bigger. Not only that, but as the energy to the pre-frontal cortex drops we manufacture far fewer new thoughts. Soon the mind is swamped by worry.

Is cortisol damage to the brain repairable?

Scientists *think* so, but research is ongoing. A large clinical study at the St Louis and Emery University is studying brain imaging to try to discover how long recovery times in humans might be. I mentioned Cushing's Disease earlier. The cortisol levels in this disease are actually caused by a pituitary tumour which drives the adrenal cortex to over produce. What we do know is after one of these tumours has been removed, it takes the effects of the cortisol a year or more to return to normal. This would indicate then that effects may, indeed, be repairable.

Allostatic Load

The term was first coined in 1993 by McEwan and Stellar when they published their findings about the effects of stress on the body. It pertains to the wear and tear your body undergoes over time when it exposed to chronic stress.

It addresses issues like changes in body type because of stress. This can be because cortisol levels are elevated in the evening, when normally they should be down making us crave different foods. The liver metabolises our food differently too, if we binge eat in the evening (another cortisol problem). Long term allostatic load leads to blood clotting and circulatory issues and, of course, heart disease.

But, why?

What is important to understand, is just like when your salary check starts to run out, you need to start borrowing, so the adrenals do the same.

Their favourite resources to plunder are the liver and the pituitary gland, which I'll get to in a moment.

The liver

I like to imagine the liver as the foreman of the body, and its effects on health are myriad. Again, this is covered in more depth in its own book *The Essential Oils Liver Cleanse.* But here are the edited highlights.

Its functions are:

- It produces bile. This helps carry away waste and break down fats in the small intestine as you digest food.
- It plays a part in producing proteins which make up blood plasma
- It produces cholesterol and other special proteins to carry fats through the body
- It converts excess glucose into glycogen to make it easier for the body to store it. (This glycogen can later be converted back to glucose for energy.)
- It regulates blood levels of amino acids. These acids form the building blocks of proteins
- It processes haemoglobin for use of its iron content (That is to say the liver stores iron.)
- It converts poisonous ammonia to urea. (Urea is one of the end products of protein metabolism which is excreted in urine.)
- It clears the blood of drugs and other poisonous substances
- It regulates blood clotting

- It builds resistance to infection by producing immune factors and removing bacteria from the blood stream

Startling isn't it? Now, cortisone is actually a glucocorticoid. That is a glucose substance originating from cholesterol which is formed in the liver. So to fulfil their need to keep producing cortisol, the adrenals take, take, take and they leech every last bit of the liver's strength.

So, consider this. How many body systems would suffer if the adrenals began to leech the livers power? I count circulation and digestion as the obvious ones, but speaking as someone who has had a blood clot in her lungs I can tell you...it threatens the entire mechanism of the body.

By the time stress has found its way to the liver, there are serious issues beginning to raise their heads.

Liver toxicity

The problem is further complicated by the fact that often our livers are in a pretty shocking state any way and may already not be working to capacity.

We live in a world of not enough. It's not only you who does not have enough time, enough money, enough internal resources generally, our entire societal structure is stretched to a point of exhaustion. This has repercussions.

Food

The farmers cannot keep up with the demand for food we need to eat, so they spray chemical fertilisers and pesticides over our food to make the harvest go further. Our bright shiny apple comes complete with heavy metal poisons which are absorbed straight into the liver.

Memory

If you listen to athletes speak of their triumphs they will often refer to muscle memory. PTSD can also show itself through muscle and memory associations. In the Mind Body Spirit we looked at Candace Pert's theory that emotions, memories and traumas become trapped within the tissues because of huge surges of neuropeptides entering cells. Many holistic practitioners believe that trauma lodges itself in the the liver, in particular.

Pharmaceutical debris

These most certainly leave their imprint. In particular, research done by my late step father, Michael Cook, showed there could be a link between a people with migraine and pethidine being used in their deliveries when they were born. Since your liver has to assimilate pharmaceutical gunk as it goes through your body, it is reasonable to assume there may be toxicity left behind.

My statistician son would demand *causation* or *correlation*? In other words, can I say that Pethidine's definitely to blame?

Not when there are drug companies with lawyers in expensive suits about no, but between you and I: the numbers are compelling.

What you also need also to be aware of is antibiotics rid the body of Vitamin B.

Lack of nutrition

Most importantly the liver depends on nutrients in the body to keep it functioning. In particular, it requires Vitamin B. At times of stress, the liver burns the vitamin too quickly and again, there is no longer enough fuel to power it

In *The Essential Oil Liver Cleanse* and then even deeper in *The Aromatherapy Eczema Treatment* I explain how toxicity here can also throw up allergies too. For the purposes of this book, it is enough for you to know that this can happen. Incidentally although the liver cleanse and allergies are the subjects of the other books, I have listed a few of the oils needed in the <u>essential oils</u> section of the book.

Pituitary Gland

The pituitary gland, again, is an endocrine player; a really important one as it goes. About the size of a pea, it is found behind the nose at the base of the brain, quite close to the optic nerves. For a long while it was thought the pituitary was the boss of the systems, but we have since found out the hypothalamus is the CEO.

The pituitary secretes many hormones, most of them related to reproduction. In women, these hormones stimulate ovulation, ripen eggs and also stimulate labour and milk when a baby has been born. In men, these hormones trigger the testes to manufacture testosterone and sperm too.

Testosterone, oestrogen and progesterone are all synthesized from cholesterol.

So now, for any of you who are seeing patients who are are struggling to conceive or have experienced any bouts of impotence, you might want to read that section again. Stress has exhausted their adrenals glands. The adrenals have leached the power from the liver for more power to make glucocorticoids. The liver can no longer produce adequate cholesterol to synthesize the sex hormones (not to mention carrying out the rest of its functions effectively.) The pituitary is no longer firing on all cylinders so sexuality, or fertility, will probably be taking a kicking. (As well as self esteem here, of course)

Interestingly, researchers recently published study into the effects of using the pharmacological version of the dance drug, *Ecstasy* (MDMA), on patients with PTSD and depression. They found that they were able activate vmPFC, which then triggered the pituitary to produce oxytocin (the neuropeptides that helps mums' bonding with new babies). They are now experimenting to try to use this to promote a feeling of emotional closeness in suffers of PTSD in a bid to speed their healing. In the blind trial in 2008, patients were given the drug alongside a series of 12 sessions of psychotherapy. Each of the subjects had already undergone six months of traditional therapy and a further three months with drugs but had shown no changes in mental state. At the end of the 12 weeks and two doses of MDMA, 92% of the patients were reported to have escaped their shell of shame and were able to recognise and resume their previous patterns of behaviour prior to their onset of the trauma.

Here then, we can see why the pituitary plays such a valuable part in our own treatments too. (Please note: I recommend you replace dance drugs with essential oils here and do not recommend taking amphetamines...just for clarity!)

Hypothalamus

He is the big boss. If you wanted to play Hannibal Lecter and get a sharp knife, you would find the hypothalamus right at the base of the brain connected to the spinal column. This location is the reason for the driving test/urgent need to urinate problem. The gland controls hunger, thirst, temperature, blood pressure, water balance and weight. The messages about anxiety go directly from the brain, down the spinal column and then affect the nerves connected to the organs. The emotions ramp up the activity of the hypothalamus sending you charging to the smallest room to reduce the amount of water in the system.

The hypothalamus is the most obvious and best recognised physical connection between the mind and the body.

Circulation

In the most simplistic terms, adrenaline forces heart rates up and up which also thickens your blood. This continuous pressure on the blood vessels eventually damages them. This can then lead to heart disease or circulation problems such as thrombosis.

Metabolic Syndrome

I just want to make a passing hat tip to Metabolic Syndrome. If this is a new term for you, it is the official term for the condition which links diabetes, high blood pressure and obesity. Scientists agree there is a complex two way interdependency between stress and metabolic syndrome.

Sufferers of metabolic syndrome are at higher risk of heart disease and strokes because of the extra pressure put on the blood vessels. Sufferers of diabetes can become very stressed by their many connected symptoms and of course, stress will exacerbate them too. According to the NHS, one in four people in the UK suffer from Metabolic Syndrome. The Asian and Afro Caribbean are especially, but not exclusively affected and it is also prevalent in patients with Polycystic Ovarian Syndrome.

Can you see how the jigsaw is starting to fit together?

To go back to the initial question of "what is stress....?"

It's trouble, and then some.

Toxicity

This is a short section for a massive learning concept. If an organ begins to dysfunction, then it will lead to toxicity.

Think of each organ in terms of their optimum working capacity of 100%. If, for instance, the adrenals drain 20% of the power of the liver, it will only have the strength to work at 80%

That leaves a "hole".

20% toxicity fills the gap.

Consider too, as the vigour of an organ wanes, it will draw from another for its life support. Like a domino effect, every system lends some capacity to sustain this cortisol problem. The more toxic the body gets, the weaker the systems become forcing them to lean on other systems and draining them too.

At every juncture, the body gets weaker and toxicity advances.

This toxicity is what leads to stress related illness such as eczema, psoriasis and migraine. Most interestingly it also activates allergic response. Again, for deeper study about this I recommend you refer to *The Essential Oils Liver Cleanse*.

Clearly though, in order to make our patients truly better, we need to eradicate this toxicity to get their organs back on an even keel.

So how do we do this? We use a many pronged approach.

Chapter 2

Yin and Yang

Chinese philosophy offers a great deal of insight into what may have happened to a body when it is stressed. Consider the body aligned to the idea of yin and yang – that is to say female and male - and the balance of energy in the body and its place in the universe.

You may have already learned some of this, as part of a way to healing, using the meridians. I use these to balance the body too, and my suggested acupressure points come in part 2 of the book.

For those of you who don't know, meridians are energy flows which run up and down the body in a North Southerly direction. There are 12 pairs of meridians and then there are also conception vessel which is yin and governing vessel which is yang and you find these at the centre of the body.

The philosophy also feels everything correlates to an element too. For instance emotions:

- Water (fear)
- Wood (anger)
- Fire (happiness)
- Earth (worry)

- Metal (grief)

Now, yin energy is moist, cool, soft and welcoming. It is passive, sustaining electromagnetic energy. It is female where yang is hard, hot masculine and active.

Yin Yang comes originally from Taoism and separates everything into these groups. However do remember to follow their flow of everything having its own energy rather than trying to put them all into a specific box.

Yin Yang is about balance at all times, but also how one can very easily fade into another. Nothing is ever entirely yin or entirely yang, more it has a tendency more to lean toward one than the other.

Think of day and night, one gradually becomes the other but there are always elements of both.

In a moment I shall talk about the relevance of yin disease but I want you to see it as its most extreme example. Taoism also subdivides elements into the following groups too: Excess and deficiency of yin and yang, internal and external stimuli, warm and cold, yin and yang and they are also further subdivided again. So, for example: *heat* - you might have warm yin and burning yang.

Yin Disease

Before I start this section I must say that I hope that Dr Laurence Wilson M.D. reads this book so I can say a well overdue thank you to him and he can see just how much it has influenced my work. Whilst the following pieces don't infringe copyright, my mind has absorbed every part of his writing on this subject, pretty much, word for word. The man is a healing genius (although often his political bias is a tad barbed). Without his website these particular insights would have been impossible over the years. He has given me personally, many jigsaw pieces to put the bits of healing knowledge together. His wisdom about vitamins and minerals, about Chinese medicine and chakra healing never fail to blow me away. I claim no part in putting the following bits together, and I would urge you to get to his website and learn so much more from him.

Stress is very much aligned to what is deemed to be Yin disease; that is: there is an excess of yin in the person. These are diseases with a colder, less energetic element to them. Patients presenting with these will have a more prevalent disposition to the following:

They have slower metabolisms and so you are likely to see some hint of a change in their weight. They may report they seem to have become more prone to fungal illnesses too. When they ail it is more likely to be because they have caught a viral infection rather than a bacterial one and so you might be looking at perpetual colds and flu.

He goes on to say:

They are more prone to parasitic organisms such as Lyme Disease or intestinal parasites for example. On a less shocking level we might be looking for headaches, complaints of premenstrual tension, breakouts of acne, painful and restricted tendon and ligament problems and ongoing yeast infections too. Cancer is also common. ***Adrenal insufficiency and adrenal burnout are your most likely indicators***.

Medically, yin also means the bodily tissues begin to lose their strength and you might find evidence they are disintegrating in some way. Yang is the more masculine, hard and dense. So with yin, you will notice a softening. Their general structure becomes weak, clearly osteoporosis would be a concern, but we might see chronic fatigue or blood problems too. Overwhelmingly the person tends to be weak, tired, depressed, anxious, and suffer the cold. For yin disease you will be looking for low thyroid activity, low adrenal activity and often low hormone levels in general. Anaemia is often found too. Incidentally the blood pertains to the element of yin.

When you meet a patient presenting with symptoms derived from an excess of yin, look back at your case history and check their age. How closely does it relate to how old they *seem*. Not only does yin present as someone who looks older, has the demeanour and outlook of someone older and potentially the bones of someone older, they will just have that sickly, worn out element to them too.

By nature we do get more yin through age. So you would expect more of these "elderly" elements to show, the blood supply becomes more rarified to the scalp and the hair can start to fall out, bones are brittle, the cold affects us more and dare I say it... we **moan!** (*At this juncture –Allow me please to remind you of the sweeping generalisations disclaimer you bought into at the start- apologies to those of our zimmer frame generation and I do appreciate what you did in the war!*)

Psychological indicators of Yin Disease

Again, bear in mind here we have this triangle of mind, body, spirit, so an emotion can make you more yin, or the high levels of yin will also influence the way you feel.

The overwhelming countenance of a person with a yin excess will be that of a victim, or more precisely "Woe is me, I am a victim", because he'll want you to know.

When yin is balanced it is passive, serene and intuitive, but think about how that would look in excess. He might feel confused and fearful and will definitely have a general front of unhappiness. There can often be episodes of deep guilt which anyone else can see is entirely unwarranted. Often they are very spacey in their demeanour and in the worst cases you can see schizoid personality traits or schizophrenia.

Dishonesty is their main tack, sometimes because they have lost a grip on reality and are confused, but often because it simply suits their means. If you were to look at a group of criminals the yin excess would present in that section of sociopaths... they are cunning, charming, they manipulate and they plot to deceive. But what about if their dishonesty comes from a different place: From fear? Do they steal to keep food on their table and might you keep hearing stories about how they walked into a door? Or, of course, you might only hear "Yes, I'm fine"; *when clearly, they're not.*

At the root of these you will usually find resentment, fervently simmering anger bubbling away. Actually, you can say activist, *or even re-activist*, because they are so worn out and have so little energy that the anger is their very driving force, it is like a catalyst to get them out of bed. This is because the hot, fierce nature of their anger is of course...yang.

You are likely to see some level of brain fog, whether that is because they are scatty, they are forgetful or even they begin to show those early signs of dementia; confusion will often rear its ugly head. In some cases the confusion may not present like that to them, but you may notice yourself trying to muddle through how they came to decisions in their thought process, you might notice their logic makes little sense. Again, I'll refer back to what I said about lies; this could be because they have become a little befuddled. Think back to what I said about people with a problem with the crown chakra in the **Mind Body Spirit of Clinical Aromatherapy**:

"It is hard to say this chakra is aligned to emotion, more a state of mind of being open, being available for intuition to enter, having a high vibration of compassion, and of sending healing goodness out into the world.

I suppose being healers we move in the right circles to see this chakra blocked open more than many other people do. This is dissociative behaviour, spiritual obsession, having your head in the clouds."

We see it again here. These people are making things up (that is their imagination is running wild), but they are disassociated or actually sometimes quite literally *away with the faeries*, because nature and magic so very much appeals.

The charm offensive too, is very yin and again we have this sociopath correlation. You don't see these as the persuaders, because these are more often *manipulators*. They draw people to them because they are enigmatic and probably have some sort of worthy cause (I'll come to that in a moment) and people like to follow. If you were to think "abuse of power" this would be emotional abuse rather than physical abuse, misdirection and twisting again. You can guarantee this person won't pull the first punch; they will provoke another into taking it.....and we are back to the victim again.

Now, I hope that most of you will go on to read *Sales Strategies for Gentle Souls* where we talk about identifying pools of potential clients. What becomes interesting here is that I suspect that most of your yin protagonists will come from one particular income stream. I'll describe this aspect and I'll let you guess why.

The Yin personality roots for the underdog, (which I referred to when I mentioned liking their causes,) mainly because they very much identify with their own position as being oppressed. You will find them fervent supporters of the welfare state. Trade unions are yin, as are institutions like the dole and DSS. Yin does not like capitalism and abhors big money corporations. Whilst the yin mind is quick and intelligent (potentially he got that clever from covering all his tracks) and knows that things like plant healing and natural energy is the best approach for him because he distrusts the quacks (his word, not mine) and this softer, floaty element to the personality will, as I said, attract him to natural healing and ancient wisdoms. However he will be very impressed by the money and trappings of the hospitals and will want a fast solution to the end of what he sees as his living hell. We are back to the element of yin: *thinks life owes him a living.* He will not want to work at healing himself because yin energy prevents him from really sticking at anything. He goes for what he deems to be a short sharp fix. What's more he will bemoan that it is his right.

I am sure you have worked out that you will find these people sitting in the doctor's waiting room moaning that they feel ill and worse still, furious that the job centre suggested they should get off their backside and go and find some work.

In their defence, you do have the chicken and egg situation that, the angrier they get, the more yin they become and then their physical symptoms also get potentially worse. The angrier they are, the more likely it is that they really *shouldn't* be at work.

What is great, of course, is if you can find a way to get a conversation with a yin person....they love the idea the earth might be able to make them better and they will not be able to contain themselves with excitement for the opportunity for their opinion to be proven right that their doctor was a fool.

Dr Wilson also gives us some really good insights into what their hormones are likely to be doing from his clinical work:

- High oestrogen levels
- Low testosterone levels
- High TSH (Thyroid)

- Sexual bonding hormones high
- Low progesterone
- High cholesterol
- Cold body temperature and of course we can say the coldness of manipulation too.

Those pointers should help you put some more essential oil ideas together.

A point which I suspect will galvanise a few thoughts. People who have an excess of yin often experiment with drugs. In particular you will see them drawn to medicinal marijuana to help them through the day. It eases their aches and pains and it allows them to hide from their depression if only for a little while. Marijuana and coffee both have elements of a mineral called cadmium which is very yang...in other words it works a bit like resentment does in projecting them through their day. Alcohol, too, holds its appeal for them, but can make them very morose.

Wilson also pointed out something which I see happening often now I know to look for it. He calls it moral relativism. That is, they skew perceptions of right and wrong, based on somebody (or something, because they often do it about animals) being the oppressed. So, for example they might jump to the defence of a homosexual or ethnic minority saying any crime they committed was acceptable because of their social position, whereas most of us would say murder is murder and rape is rape regardless of the background of the perpetrator.

You might also notice the slogan they carry round with them: "All you need is love", completely oblivious to how normal people translate this into everyday life. They can't see past meditate and everything will be good. Actually I hadn't thought of it until I wrote it but they then continue with this expectation that someone else will take care of them. Again, they renege on their responsibilities to themselves. Instead of the welfare state will provide this time we have "The *universe* will provide". (Incidentally I whole heartedly agree that it *will* provide, the difference is I am working my ass off to give it a hand... and that's yang energy).

Lastly, notice how the yin person talks about people and animals "I'd take animals over people any day". You are likely to see campaigning for animals rights etc too. The people who let animals out of labs and stop the Grand National starting are all potential clients ripe for the taking. Again they are battling for the underdog but they are also giving capitalists pigs the finger for an extra kick.

So then, how did they get this way?
Heavy metals, fertilisers, petrochemicals, pharmaceutical debris, radioactivity and electromagnetic fields are all yin.

Read that again.

So now, let's think this out.

We know all of the food we are eating is sprayed unless we eat organic. We take antibiotics in particular for myriad conditions like candida / thrush which is a yeast infection and can often have a parasitic source (*see The Aromatherapy Eczema Treatment*.) We are less than a hundred years since a nuclear bomb and we are ENTIRELY surrounded by wireless technology. (Incidentally if you want to know more about the dangers of that see *The Essential Oil Liver Cleanse*.)

There's more, and this is a little scarier, but we will address it in the diet section.

Fruit is yin, so is raw food and also any food that is fermented like yoghurt or tofu. Sugars refined or otherwise, alcohol and milk... all yin.

Drugs: Marijuana, cocaine and other amphetamines are yin.

Hmmm, that's more than a little yin!

Clearly women will be more susceptible to yin because it is the moist feminine energy, but also our actual chemical make-up differs in that women have high levels of yin copper and men more yang zinc.

Vitamin C is yin, so if someone has been habitually supplementing, then they will have an excess of yin. An excess of yin will also indicate there is a residue of other old female minerals lying dormant and raising toxicity in their systems too. Again I'll come back to that in the vitamin therapy section.

How I originally found this wisdom of learning was when I first became ill with a pulmonary embolism. It happened just 5 weeks after going on a plane and although I did not present with thrombosis the clot very quickly moved to my lungs. Air travel is yin. Air, itself, is yin as well as the process of moving away from the earth and blood is yin. When your liver is deficient (remember the liver is responsible for the formation of plasma) it takes on a yin bias. In the *Essential Oil Liver Cleanse* we address this in far more depth, but here, know that anger will be the worst protagonist to make this happen.

From an astrological point of view, we are in a very yin time. The Age of Aquarius is about connecting, whether that might be through the grace of God... or by email!

Sexual activity is yin that would be thinking about it, doing it or even simulating it; these are all yin. I suppose, again, we can say this is connecting. Since we mention it the very thought of it does knacker me out. Maybe that's the reason! Husband of mine, that headache I have been complaining about...it's all down to yin!

Most depressing of all, too much bathing is apparently yin – but that isn't going to deter me!

Note to self: You are clearly getting FAR too old and yin. It seems a bath is more fun than sex! PS I have also noticed you are growing increasingly far too excited about chocolate being yang!

I'll come back in a moment and talk about the energy centres but, in the spirit of balance, I'll just quickly cover yang disease.

Wilson used a very clever analogy that helped me with this. Think of Rome. It started off as this beautiful ideal, but then as time went on it became crueller more dominating and dictatorial. This is the energy of yang. It also demonstrates how energy can change with too much of one thing. On the flipside of the yin soul in the doctor's waiting room, might you find this one on a sales team? Or would he burn out the yang and become more yin? Depends when you catch him I suppose.

So, first of all, you will probably notice the yang shape. They get that stocky, thick-set look. They are macho, big and brutal. If a person has gone too yang - they become dictatorial and cruel. You are not as likely to this person as a stress patient because they have lost touch with their feelings, they are still extremely or overly rational and they will have no perception of their effects on other people.

In other words, yang means you really don't feel sorry for yourself and therefore even if there are some organic symptoms of stress, they are far too self-centred and driven, at this point, to perceive them. People who have an excess of yang have no fear and certainly would never feel victimised because this would mean they would have to accept they have given up control. They are driven risk-takers and have immense energy. Often they are racists.

You will not see these presenting with sexual worries because actually, for them, sex is not about desire, it is more about burning off energy or in some cases exerting power. There is no reason for them to worry about performance at this point. Of course, if the hormonal balance starts to betray them, then we know the energy is turning yin. They are beginning to soften. Again I think it is really weird how we already say these things anyway. If a woman goes off sex because she has become too yin, she is cold: she is frigid. A man loses his yang hard erection, yes, he goes soft.

The line

So where is the line? At what point does a person become TOO yin or too yang. Who can say? It almost feels like political alliances doesn't it? You have the far left communist radicals who dream of a Marxist ideal and then on the extreme right you have the fascist dictators. So, one would suppose the rest of us are sitting on the fence, really, tagging the healthy line (how very Liberal party of us!)

What we *do* know, is when the energy becomes too far towards yin, you are about to see an insidious breakdown of health. Depression most certainly is looming and chronic illness is likely to follow.

The following list (adapted from Taichido.com) will hopefully inspire you to come up with your own dynamic ways of healing. On looking at each client individually, I think you find you draw some incredible conclusions about whether they lean more to yin than yang...incidentally note that the seasons could be having an impact too.

Yin	Yang
Female	Male
Cold	Hot
Damp	Dry
Soft	Hard
Amorphous	Formed
Artistic	Scientific
Autumn / Winter	Spring/Summer
Black	White
Body	Mind
Centripetal	Centrifugal
Child	Parent

Chronic	Acute
Completion	Incipience
Constant pain	Intermittent pain
Containing	Bursting
Contraction	Expansion
Dark	Light
Death	Life
Deep	Surface
Deep pain	Superficial pain
Diffusion	Focus
Down	Up
Earth	Sky / Air
Form	Space
Front	Back
Fruits	Grains
Gathering energy	Expending energy
Green	Red
Hell	Heaven
Inclusive	Exclusive
Inertia	Effort
Inside of limbs	Outside of limbs
Interior	Exterior
Internal	External
Introvert	Extrovert
Leafy vegetable	Root vegetable

Lower body	Upper body
Mass	Individual
Material	Immaterial
Moon	Sun
More intellectual	More physical
Mother	Father
Nature	Technology
Negative	Positive
Night	Day
North	South
Pain does not move	Pain moves around
Parasympathetic	Sympathetic
Passive	Active
Past	Future
Proton	Electron
Receptive	Assertive
Relaxation	Tension
Responsive	Aggressive
Rest	Movement
Right side	Left side
Roots	Branches
Sensation	Conceptualization
Sinking	Rising
Spoon	Knife
Stomach	Head

Structure	Function
Supporting	Supported
Synthesis	Analysis
Tradition	Change
Transporting organs	Storage organs
Water	Fire
Wet	Dry
Yielding	Resistance

Yin organs	Yang organs
Transform and store qi blood, bodily fluids and essence	Separates impure substances from the food and then excrete them.
Lungs	Stomach
Spleen	Small intestine
Heart	Large intestine
Liver	Urinary bladder
Kidneys	Gall gladder
	Triple burner

Energy centre performances

Right now let's go back to the chakras and go over what you might expect to see.

If you have not already read it, the fundamentals of how the chakras connect the emotions to the physical body are covered, at length in the *Mind Body Spirit of Clinical Aromatherapy*.

Yin people are no longer grounded (*going out of their minds* and potentially are *off their 'eads!*) Notice their root chakra, is it working effectively? Or is the sacral chakra over compensating for it? Is the crown spinning out control? You might even notice these spinning very fast in the opposite direction to the others. Most of all I would suspect some disturbance at the solar plexus, at least.

Yang chakra patterns by contrast are over developed and very open at the root and numbers two and three. They have no leanings towards love, companionship and compassion so four and five are less used, six and seven are potentially redundant (although you can be sure yang insisted no severance pay!)

An interesting insight is into the cultural differences of prayer between Christianity and earth religions and how that affects energy. Christianity draws energy from heaven, whereas most holistic medicine predominately draws sustenance from the earth. Moving energy upwards through the body is yin, whereas down is more yang. Clearly when teaching meditation to people in this state we should teach energy in through the crown and then harness them at the root. We want to ground them by anchoring them back in reality.

A reminder: there was a chakras chart with *Mind Body Spirit*. *F*or ease, you can find it again at:

https://buildyourownreality.leadpages.co/chart/

I find it useful to print one of these off, each week, to scribble patient's notes on and compare how the activity of each chakra changes through each week of their treatment.

Summing Up

A recap: Originally the term stress was an engineering term for how an object reacted to pressure. In your clinic then, patients potentially have become so stressed they are no longer able to Fight and Flight, so they flee.... and potentially they can go right out of their minds.

In short, they are not stressed. They are fundamentally broken.

So how then, do we fix them?

Part 2

Chapter 3 The Medicine

Now if you are all excited because you have found the key to healing every person suffering with stress, I am about to bring you to a screaming, smashing and rather unsettling halt.

Plant medicine is yin.

Ah!

But, some essential oils are more yin than others. Top and top-middle notes are your worst protagonists. If you think about it, it makes sense. We need to ground stressed patients with slow, earthy, warm base notes.

There is a list of which are the good and the not so good oils in the essential oils section.

We do have a secret weapon at our disposal. Clue: it is something that is very yang. It is hard, dry, hot, and exciting.

Enough with your yin phallic debauchery! The secret weapon is minerals. The dense, hard calcium and the bright, excitable magnesium, for instance. Vitamin therapy is very yang. We also have food and then we also have our varying ways of balancing the subtle bodies and cleaning the systems with oils.

First, let's look at the methods and then lastly we will look at oils.

The steps are:

- Soothe the mind and get them to sleep
- Cleanse the body
- Nourish the body
- Release the Spirit

Now clearly in therapy you are likely to be tackling two or three aspects all at once. How to write these in the correct order has become a constant source of annoyance to me in this book. Therefore then, I am opting to cover them in the order of looking after the mind and spirit first, then the body last, simply because it seems easiest to write it this way. As the therapist it is your job to treat what you deem to be the most pressing aspect of your patient's illness first.

Before you do anything...

Psychically protect yourself. (Covered in *Complete Guide to Clinical Aromatherapy and Essential Oils of the Physical Body*)

Please get into the habit of putting a really strong physical protection around you when you are seeing clients and the moment they leave, rinse your aura down. These are poorly people, physically and spiritually, they need extra life force to sustain them, they will not even realise they are draining your of yours.

Just in the same way you are teaching them to balance themselves, you must ensure you are grounded. By all means be a transmitter of healing energy,(in fact, you *must* be that,) but for goodness sake don't take on any of their c**p and hold on to your own too.

Understanding the gender distinction of stress

Physiologically we know that men and women's minds react differently to stress, but psychologically we don't know why.

We do know that men tend to stress more about things which affect their ego or identity. In driving simulation studies for instance, they react more to the stress than women who aren't that bothered by that kind of "fail".

Studies have also shown that women who have to stand up and speak in front of people react less to stress if they have a supportive spouse besides them. Further, they are more soothed by having another woman with them there.

What I found out in my research into the amygdala is women process fear differently. In a clinical trial where subjects watched a horror film opposite amygdalae were lit: left in women and right in men. Scientists think this might have something to do with why us gal's remember everything ever said in an argument when men are simply able to move on. The right amygdala is responsible for taking action and so it also might explain why a bloke is more likely to clout someone threatening them, when we birds might opt to try to talk it out. What was more interesting was when a group of gay men were tested, their brains lit up in the same way as the girls.

What this is going to mean, then, is the source of the stress, and the reaction to the stress, will be different in men than it is from women.

Always keep in mind that outward symptoms in the physical body are clues and pointers to what is going on in a person's head. Certain emotions affect specific organs and often the same root cause can be seen over and over in health. It its simplest form:...a person dying of a broken heart.

Sometimes these are very easy to tease out, others will need a bit more coaxing.

Your first tool is always to be listening. Even if the words are not being said "I hate my work" or "My wife is a harpee," general tone and responses to your case history investigations should obviously give some clues. Remember you're the empath; learn to try to read between the lines. There is no need to comment, simply store away your information and then choose oils aligned to their clues.

From there, I would suggest you consult the back.

Massage
When you massage your patient, you will be well used to listening to your fingers to find where the knots of stress hide. The tissues of the back more than any, can you give you clues as to underlying dis-tress.

Just as the reflexes on the feet are like a map of the organs of the body, so the back is a treasure map for the seekers of the true source of stress.

The shoulder mantle is the classic place for work stress to lodge. From a postural aspect of sitting in front of a computer to the defensive stance in front of the boss, the shoulders curl in, they clench and they tighten.

Money, of course, influences many of our lives. This is a particular problem in men. The deeply ingrained need to provide for their family can often work as a negative driver for many sufferers of stress.

The thoracic parts of the back (the long run down over the ribs) and also the pelvic regions will often be very tight.

Relationship aspects of stress will betray themselves in the pelvic area and also the backs of the thighs.

You should need very little help with these relaxing oils but if you do, you can find them here.

The spiritual aspect is far too personal to dissect in theory. Everyone's challenges are their own and they are myriad. I feel though, very strongly that a key element is often we move to far away from the path God intended for us. Yes, that can, certainly, be morally, but it is not my place to judge or it even could be the way someone expresses their relationship to their faith...whatever that may be.

One thing I find, though, is many people become stressed because they no longer find joy in their lives. Life comes about washing and ironing and earning a buck. For my mother in law this is heaven because she loves cleaning but that's not the same for every soul (least of all for me!)

If you can find a way for the patient to tap into something that they love, something that gives them a reason to get up in the morning; that is a powerful tool.

Whilst we can alleviate the effects of the stress, we can do nothing about its source and, in fact, that will come back over and over again. Some might suggest the person is facing some kind of karmic lesson.

We have the oils at our disposal to give the patient a gentle nudge or even a great big kick in the right direction, but ultimately their best healing is going to come from their own inner work.

The chakras will give you insights to possible forces at play. Use oils to balance the "offending chakras" and you should expect the emotions and spiritual issues to start to come into alignment.

You can find the chakra oils here:

From my own experience, there is nothing more healing than quiet. Circumstances changed my life forever in 2009 when my husband and I both lost our jobs and it lead to having to sell our home. The funny thing was, with nothing left to lose, we could make choices with no other concerns in mind and we decided to get out of the city.

Being alone with your thoughts

Have you noticed just how much people affect your thinking? Whether you read, hear people talking or even watch others doing *stuff* it affects you way you think. If there is a way you can get your patient to take some time out away from everything, I think it would really help. Whether that is away from work or away from everyone is going to be their call. Going to the quiet for me meant no more phone calls, no more explaining what I was doing to people but most of all no more noise. More than anything, this is what has healed *me*.

It's amazing what you find out about yourself when you just take time to listen!

Brainwaves

For many stress related complaints, from blood pressure to angina, the doctor will prescribe beta blockers. These are designed to calm the nerve impulse transmitters which increase heart beat. What is interesting is, when we are very alert, our mind operates on a beta wavelength too.

Beta

This is the fastest of all the brain waves at 14-40 hz. This is the seat of logic, or learning and focus. This is a very useful state. Problems start though, when the brain is unable to slip from this fast cycling to go to a slower state. This leads to insomnia, restlessness and all other symptoms related to stress.

Alpha

This is slower and you will notice in comparison to beta has a smaller gap, being only between 7.5-14hz. This is light meditation and day dreaming, on the whole. It is that blissful sigh of relief when you close your eyes, lying on the grass in the sun. This is the gateway to the subconscious. Clearly as you take your mind closer to 7.5 hz, intuition comes stronger.

Theta

In deep mediation or light sleep, theta waves kick in. Intuition is at its strongest at the 7-8 border, and then visualisation becomes very powerful. This is the wavelength where you will recognise REM sleep.

Many of you will know this is when our thoughts are at their most powerful and we can bring about great change. More importantly in this state there seems to be a break in the boundaries between the realities and it is here where we feel most at one with the universe.

Delta

For the most of us, this is deep dreamless sleep, although for the clever flyers amongst you this is also achieved in transcendental meditation (I wonder if the electrodes anchored them down?!). From a health, and certainly a healing point of view, this is the most valuable "holiday" for the mind. Doing everything you can to help your patient achieve deep sleep is the very best way to restore your patient. It, potentially, may have a single bigger effect than anything else you prescribe.

Gamma

Recently scientists have realised there is a, rarely seen, length at 40hz where the brain exhibits gamma waves. This is the state of bliss and we are told it can only be achieved through meditation.

Now what is interesting is that people who meditate regularly, tend to have a resting brain wave at the frequency of alpha, a significantly calmer and more constructive state than everyone elses' beta. So the key, then, to stilling the mind has got to be practice, practice, practice. With that though come the benefits of reduction of stress, insights into potential life problems and creative manifestation of ways to solve them.

Hypnosis

I am not very good at meditation, my mind chatters too much. I have found hypnosis to be far more help to me. I have used normal hypnosis and past life regression to bring about amazing results. What I find extremely useful is this is guided work at a very low cost.

By accessing the theta waves very quickly, I find it to be like opening a book. I simply access the index to see what I want to find out and then go straight to the page. I love how relaxed I feel after the work and I find it helps me sleep better too.

From a physiological stand point you can use hypnosis in exactly the same way as essential oils. You can ramp up testosterone and reduce insulin by simply resetting the trigger settings in the brain.

Hypnosis addresses *specific* issues very quickly and efficiently. I think addressing your patients fundamental self esteem issues alongside their need to switch off and rest is an amazing starting point for your healing. Re-enforced by essential oils, this is an incredibly powerful tool. In the free book *The Complete Guide to Clinical Aromatherapy and Essential Oils* there is a free download for them to access and start using alongside your therapy.

For ease, you can download this at **https://buildyourownreality.leadpages.co/hypnother apy-mp3/**

However, it is worthwhile encouraging them to download *The Complete Guide* not only to access the download themselves but also to get a finer understanding of what aromatherapy can do for them.

Mark Bowden is an amazing hypnotherapist and I am extremely grateful to him for doing this for me. I use his recordings myself and I call him "Master of the Mind". In just a few short days I find great results from listening to his downloads.

Mark has very cleverly created a system of downloads which can tap into virtually any aspect of the stress you might encounter. This free download will help your clients to learn to trust this choice of therapy. Normally Mark's downloads retail at around £11 so this is a fantastic add on service for your clients. His details can be found in the directory of the other book.

It is worth encouraging your clients to have a go at this, if for no other reason, than to calm them to sleep. By all means use the download yourself, in fact I recommend it. Incidentally, in the chakra's section of the *Mind Body Spirit* I talk about how the root chakra can affect your attitudes to money and where it is a good or bad thing.

"In particular this [root chakra] might relate to limiting beliefs about money, or even about advancement in general. In the most extreme example, we have all seen money turn some people into right nasty pieces of work...but what if, as a

child you began to believe this was the only thing money could do. I can tell you now, that child will never grow into a person who is able to earn a decent living, because his own conscience tells him it bad.

Since this perception of reality is ultimately one of the main things that stands in the way of whether a hardworking person becomes a successful wealthy person, you might want to address this....and Mark would certainly be the man to help you. He'll undo that idea in a jiff and I bet you.... money will start flowing to your hands.

CBT

These days CBT or Cognitive Behavioural Therapy is the darling of the medical profession. They recognise how effective reframing clients' thoughts can be.

What you will find is since many of your patient's perceive themselves to be the victim; they cannot see their part in the process of regaining control. By teaching them strategies to rethink every day stressors, their lives can be completely transformed.

I would recommend this qualification as a valuable source of CPD. Otherwise I would suggest this is a time for referral to trusted colleague.

Counselling and Psychotherapy

When you are using essential oils well, you move the mind and spirit along. They can also uncover long forgotten memories and traumas which are causing patient's disease. If you suspect this is the case, get a business card out of your purse and refer to a qualified counsellor so they can help them work through the process.

Incidentally I should add here, these referrals go *alongside* your therapy, they do not replace them. The oils will continue to do their jobs and reveal clues as to the problems which may lurk.

For some people, the root of their stress may have held them together like sticky tape for a very long time. When they finally fall apart, it can be a complex set of emotions. Remember what you know about PTSD, the amygdala holds onto the memory and processes it sometimes a long time after the event. Often these memories won't come to the surface until the brain knows that the danger has actually passed. The fact the memory comes up with you might be seen as a compliment about how safe they feel. Repay that with the respect of finding them the best help available to them.

Watch, observe, but unless you are qualified, do not counsel. That is someone else's job.

Chapter 4

Detoxifying The Physical body

Ok so we start by cleansing the liver and supporting the adrenals. Again, The Essential Oil Liver Cleanse will help you better with this as it has more oils included but the best oils to use are:

Liver: Rosemary, carrot, eucalyptus

Adrenals: Mandarin and camomile

Pituitary: Best helped with nutmeg.

Oils to remove toxicity

Your best oil to get rid of fertilisers and organic pesticides is Oakmoss Resin. This oil now has restrictions on it since there were some desensitisation issues in the perfume industry. It can no longer be used in dilutions in excess of 0.1%.

Benzoin, angelica and amber oils are the best oils for removing pharmaceutical debris.

Lemon verbena removes peroxides. (For example: chlorine in sanitary wear).

Positive Ions (fluorescent bulbs, vdu emissions) - Cypress

Heavy metals – Citronella

Radiation – Garlic

For those who want to go elbow deep, even further into this gunk, I have gone more deeply and added a more full oils list in *The Essential Oil Liver Cleanse*.

I would also take time to ensure that you stimulate acupressure points to ensure the oils move toxins, but the body actually physically chucks them out too. It is far more effective and it will encourage the patient's body to work with your oils.

Acupressure Points

The acupressure points are located along meridians of the body. These are energy flows which traverse the body from head to toe. In total there are twelve pairs and also a yin governing vessel and yang conception vessel which run along the entire of the body and regulate all of the other pairs. The vital life force chi or (Qi) runs continually along them. If, however, a blockage stops the flow then toxicity arises and disease begins to form.

The organs, through the body, are seen as having a predominately male or hot and active energy, or a feminine, cool, passive and moist energy. Male organs are small intestine, large intestine, triple warmer, bladder, stomach and the gall bladder. Female organs are: lung, kidney, spleen, heart, circulation and the liver.

Using these points along the meridians helps to clear blockages and triggers certain organs to alleviate the affects of stress. Integrate them into your massage or encourage your patient to apply their homecare treatments over them. These points work like floodgates for toxins. They remove any blockages so optimum healing can begin. When you locate the correct point, apply pressure for about 30 seconds to clear it.

Whilst it is advisable to do this daily, it is also important to remember meridian work is a very powerful tool in its own right, even without the essential oils. Therefore there must also be a mindfulness not to over-stimulate.

There are diagrams of the respective meridians to help you at **https://buildyourownreality.leadpages.co/vitamins/**

In particular we use the meridian for the liver and also the kidneys to cleanse the system of toxicity. Again, because this pertains to the liver, I have put far more acupressure points in that book but three very good ones for cleansing the stress from each organ are:

LV2 – Xing Jian- This is found on the left leg, on the top of the foot. It is located between the bones of the big and second toes, in line with the fork which connects the toes. Measure one finger width away from the fork to find the point.

Apply pressure down and slightly pointed towards the bones of the second toe. The acute discomfort is the sensation of it clearing and emptying.

LV4 – Zhong Feng – Located on the rear of the ankle bone in the nook of the Achilles tendon.

This point is to bring more heat to the liver and alleviate stagnation.

LV6 Xi Guan – This one *hurts*! Inside of the leg, by the side of the knee at the very source of the calf muscle

KD4 – Da Zhong- Found on the inside of the leg at the back of the ankle

KD3 – Tai Xi- Just a little bit up from KD4, this is found just above the ankle

KD6- Zhao Hai At the front of the ankle

Using the detoxifying oils shown in the toxicity section, particularly on these points will greatly enhance your healing.

Water

I shouldn't have to write this, but I know if I don't there will be trouble. Please ensure your patient is drinking copious amounts of water to flush these toxins through. I am sure most of you are aware of the effects of drinking to little anyway. Spaciness, headaches, joint pain, difficult thinking straight, constipation and dry skin...and the list goes on. *Please* get them to drink plenty of water. Your results will be far better.

Chiropractic Indicators and Concerns

There is an excellent chart to go with this section. It contains all the main misalignments that chiropractors treat to put the spine straight.

Download it at:

https://buildyourownreality.leadpages.co/chiropract ic/

I think you will find it a useful addition to your case histories.

You might also find that some of your organic dysfunction stems from a misalignment in the spine. In fact, this is very often the case. Every nerve in the body (except for the olfactory nerves which traverse the sinuses) runs through the spinal column. So, then, a straight spine is vitally important to health. You also know that the aura and chakras, which connect the physical body to the spiritual body, also run through the spine.

Should a vertebra become misaligned, then it will lean on a nerve. When a nerve gets pinched it sends stress signals, and thus toxicity, along to its corresponding organs. Actually more specifically...it releases cortisol.

I address this more fully in *The Aromatherapy Eczema Treatment* but here, most relevantly, you may find resonance with the occurrence of headaches when you are stressed.

In particular here, the cervical vertebrae (C1, C2, C3) can confuse the brain into transferred pain. These cervical vertebrae share nerve tracts with the brain. Strangely though, the brain has no way of discerning the difference between pains in the neck or the head, and so it translates these sensations as a headache.

It can be hard to visualise just how easily a spine becomes misaligned and, actually, even bad posture can make it happen. I sink into one hip, leaning on one leg, when I am standing for any period of time. This is a classic problem. The tendons shorten and the pelvis actually starts to lean to that side.

Another bad problem is carrying your bag on your shoulder. Having all that excess weight on one side will force your shoulder down over time.

The problem is that if there is a shoulder out, the opposite hip will often try to compensate for it and you get this click, click, click as the spine gradually becomes crooked.

Get your patient to stand straight in front of you with their feet a little bit a part. Ask them to put their thumbs on their hip bones. Do their thumbs look like they are in alignment to you?

Stand behind them. Does their shoulder mantle look straight? If not, a chiropractor referral is incredibly important. It is impossible for you to achieve optimum vitality if the spine is not straight.

Exercise

I'm not sure how much to write here because I don't think there will be any surprises. Of course, it helps to get your patient moving, if only to get them to expend more energy to get them to sleep! The benefits of exercise are countless, feel better look better and actually be better! Serotonin levels surge and, clearly, it will do a lot to get the yin constitution body warm too.

Aggressive exercise is yang, where a tranquil walk or yoga is yin. I do however feel the benefits outweigh the "risks" of adding to the yin overload here. I think it is worth saying that exercising too rigorously releases more cortisol whereas moderate exercise counters it.

By the far the best recommendation I can give about exercise is:

Get your patient active; find them something they like to do, and something they are likely to stick at. Really, they need to make the recommendations and put the hard work in themselves with this one.

Revitalising the body

Some of this will be obvious. We ideally need to try and wean our patients off the dietary crutches they may be using. Caffeine becomes a no-no. If needs be, replace with decaf, and the same applies for tea.

Fizzy drinks, or worse still those caffeinated ones which make you want to fight the world - lose them! Alcohol, being a stimulant should go, and most of all sugar. I shall also add here, even though it tastes like you are eating dust, in my opinion, whole grains are far better than processed white flour products when treating patients for stress.

Again here, I will press the urgency for drinking more water.

Diet

As we are cleaning the body, we need to both move the debris from the gut but also give the body a well earned rest. The majority of the 21st century food is overly refined and also laden with the heavy metals which enabled the retailers to get them to the optimum number of tables.

Don't get me wrong, no one falls for the allure of the bright green apple more than me! Worst still was the red apple until I gave one a really good scrub once and all the waxing came off! I am very lucky to have an orchard of apple trees in my garden but, since I like making apple cakes and crumbles far too much for them to last all year, I do fall for the supermarket tricks quite often too.

Organic is always going to be better (or home grown is best) but it comes at a price tag which some can ill afford. So what I will say is this. Eating fresh fruit and vegetables is the most important thing. If going organic is going to be prohibitive...never mind. We have tools at our disposal to sort that out. Having said that: if you are shopping for taste, metal-free always tastes better, hands down.

Short Term Stress

I'll address this one first, because it is the easier diet to get your head round. However, the chances are that by the time a patient is referred to you for stress, their constitution will be in a pretty shocking state. You should, for people who are weakened by stress, choose the diet for long term.

Short term stress might be after a driving test, or a set of exams I suppose, everyone will be different.

For this we want to clear the system in a short sharp shock. We do this by putting the patient on a fresh fruit and veg detox. The first 48 hrs should be fruit juices and water only. I have to say I have never managed more than one day, mainly because of the amount of complicated washing up my juicer requires! Some people go longer; four days would be the absolute max.

After that period, introduce raw and cooked vegetables and whole grains. This fits very well with the Ayurvedic principles which I shall address more in a moment.

Long Term Stress

This is more complex and although I have put them into separate sections I suggest you read it in conjunction with the section on vitamins and minerals.

If you think back to your lessons about digestion you may remember learning about amino acids which are the building blocks for life? What's more most of the foods recommended in it are predominately yang.

There are two types of amino acids, these are essential and non-essential. The essential acids isoleucine, leucine, lysine, methionine, phenylalanine, threonine, tryptophan and valine *should* be synthesised through diet. The problem is if there is too much toxification in the liver from heavy metals et al, they can no longer do that.

Since amino acids play a large part in immunity, cell regeneration healthy skin, hair and nails, we can see how stress may also make us look not so great! They also help your body to produce vital enzymes and hormones, including insulin and glucagon that help regulate blood sugar and stop you storing excess fat, so again we can see an obvious link there too.

So for the most part we are looking at choosing foods which will help them to rebuild these amino acids and also supplementing them to give them a boost too.

The best food type for this is red meat. Ideally, you should aim to have 3 servings a day for three weeks. If that seems too heavy, go for two and some white meat too. Remember it need not be beef, it could be bacon, pork, ham, venison, game etc

Now, unfortunately this diet will be contraindicated in 2 groups. The first is obvious, those who do not eat meat. The second is those people who have liver disease, rather than dysfunction, so things like hepatitis, cirrhosis etc. Their bodies do not process amino acids in the same way and so leave recommendations about their diet squarely at the doctor's door.

For those who do not eat meat, I suggest three good portions of legumes a day. These are excellent sources of protein and do not have the fat concerns of meat.

As an overview, your predominately yang foods are drying warming and dense. They are, what I would term as, winter warming foods. We are looking at meat, eggs, grains, potatoes, root veg, warming spices, salt, cheese, garlic, onions and ginger.

Vitamin therapy

We know vitamins and minerals are vital on a number of fronts. Your patients system is in a state of collapse so we have to nourish it. They are potentially in a state of yin overdrive and this yang element will help to counter it.

You should have surmised, by now, vitamin B is top of the list, because its supplies are depleted in the liver. Prescribe a Vitamin B Complex to cover the whole gamut of healing possibilities it can provide.

There is more. Vitamin B cannot be absorbed without adequate amounts of vitamin C. This should also be prescribed. Be aware of the varying degrees of quality in the brands you use. I have always used Natures Own and Nutri-West. To understand how minerals work, consider them as working in pairs on an axis. If one becomes depleted, the other one rockets up – rather like a seesaw. This is oversimplified as in fact all of them are interdependent on each other. In actual fact, the interaction is far more complex as some complement each other and others aggravate, but for the purposes of this, my rendition works.

A far clearer version of this diagram is available at **https://buildyourownreality.leadpages.co/vitamins/**

for you to print off and use in your consultations with your clients.

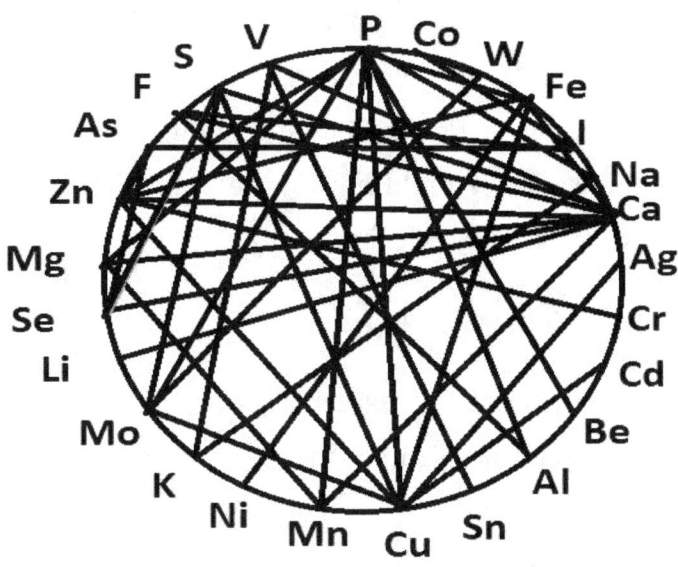

Ag Silver	F Fluorine	Ni Nickel
Al Aluminim	Fe Iron	P Phosphorus
As Arsenic	Hg Mercury	S Sulphur
Be Beryllium	I Iodine	Se Selenium
C Carbon	K Potassium	Sn Tin
Ca Calcium	Li Lithium	V Vanadium
Cd Cadmium	Mg Magnesium	W Tungsten
Co Cobalt	Mn Manganese	Zn Zinc
Cr Chromium	Mo Molybdenum	
Cu Copper	Na Sodium	

Magnesium

I'm going to get on my soapbox now in campaign for my beloved magnesium. A bit of background is, when I was carrying my last child I suffered a blood clot in my lungs. I was given a drug called Clexane which stripped all the calcium from my blood. No-one told me to take calcium supplements which, I now know, they should have done. This affected my already depleted levels of magnesium.

Some symptoms of depleted magnesium are:

Tics, muscle spasms, cramps, restless legs, seizures, anxiety, and irregular heart rhythms migraine headaches, insomnia, depression, and chronic fatigue, amongst others. It can also be a source of problems for incontinence issues too. Many experts suspect magnesium may in fact be the key to Metabolic Syndrome.

The tell tale sign for me was my husband's biggest complaint in life. I am a massive fidget in bed. I have restless legs and as I am falling asleep, I jump very aggressively and suddenly. Then I read this was a classic sign of magnesium deficiency. I couldn't believe it! But yes, after just a few days of supplementing no more restless legs or jumping when I fall asleep. Not only that, no more PMT or migraines either.

What's more, when he was finally born, the child was a dreadful sleeper. I mean waking twenty or thirty times every night. The first night he slept through, he was aged four. A week earlier I started him on a children's supplement of magnesium. His concentration is better and his behaviour is very much improved. I deliberately left out an aspect of how a person becomes very yin. It is not likely to be genetically passed from mother to child, but it is definitely congenital. The same applies to magnesium deficiency. That is, to say: because my condition became so extreme when he was in utero, he was born the same way.

Magnesium people! It's the future!

And, actually, it makes sense because magnesium in fruit develops when it reaches maturity. What do we know about fruit retailing now? They pick food too early. Magnesium is naturally found in the largest quantities in leafy green vegetables, nuts, oily fish, fruit then whole grains. Strangely too, when you cook leafy greens, the magnesium efficiency increases too, same for grains and fruits.

How magnesium absorbs and is assimilated is important because people who experience large bouts of diarrhoea will not be able to assimilate it; the body's natural response is to expel it. So for people who present with problems such as IBS or Crohns, for instance, you should administer in a different manner. Magnesium is better absorbed through the skin. Prescribe Epsom salts baths or magnesium chloride oil (which isn't actually an oil at all more a serum) for far better results.

The recommended daily allowance is 400mg per day so I prescribe 300 with the hope the rest will come from improved diet. Should we have misjudged and have prescribed too much then the body naturally dispels it through diarrhoea

Calcium

You will notice from the chart that calcium (Ca) and magnesium (Mg) sit on opposite lines. This is because they are wholly inter dependant on each other. You may remember from your chemistry lessons that elements are either positively or negatively charged. In the case of mg and Ca, they are both divalent cations (which, translated means they both have a double positive charge). What this means is they compete for absorption in the body. The higher the level of calcium, the harder it is for the magnesium to absorb.

On the surface then, it looks like you should not supplement calcium. However between the ages of 30-35 a person loses the ability to store calcium and so after that age, yes, it *is* advisable to do so. Since the calcium/ magnesium balance has a direct bearing on production of D3 aim for a supplement of this too. Deficiency of D3 is thought to be a contributory factor in the development of many strains of cancer.

Zinc

Stress decreases zinc which in turn causes copper levels to rise. Do you recall I said women have more copper naturally and men more zinc? Likewise copper is yin and zinc is yang. Jigsaw pieces....

Zinc is actually responsible for over a 100 different processes in the body but, again, edited highlights. It has a calming effect on the brain. If you have an upsurge in copper, mood cannot be stabilised. Low zinc is found in patients with depression, most notably those with post natal depression. There is also a hypothesis being tested that zinc may also affect serotonin uptake.

It also affects the thyroid. It plays a contributory part in the production of TRH by the hypothalamus which controls how your thyroid gland works. Ironically the lifespan of TRH is only about 2 minutes as it only goes a matter of inches in the blood stream before it is broken down. Without it though, the thyroid cannot regulate itself.

Now, in some ways we will be damaging zinc *ourselves* in this treatment so again it is important to supplement. Phytates in whole grains, rice corn and legumes all impede absorption of zinc and since this is a large part of the prescribed diet, this needs to be replaced. (You can't do right for doing wrong, can ya?)

Amino Acids
When a person is severely depleted they may show symptoms which could be mistaken for hypoglycaemia. They go light

headed and can feel disoriented and generally weak. To stop this happening, prescribe Core Level Health Reserve and Amino All by Nutri West. Neither of these should be taken during pregnancy or if there is a high likelihood of becoming pregnant.

Sodium /Potassium

The balance of sodium and potassium is complicated and is connected to the balance of calcium-magnesium. If those have been off kilter, like a seesaw, these will be too.

In stages of acute stress (remember we are aligning this to short term stress) the ratio is likely to be high sodium/ low potassium but by the time stress has become chronic the ratio shifts to low sodium / high potassium.

Now at first glance it might seem intuitive to add more salt to your cooking, but there are more disadvantages than advantages to this. At the very basest level prescribe a multi-vitamin/ mineral to boost the sodium levels. With the magnesium addressed this should be enough to bring it the ratios pretty much into alignment.

Chapter 5 The essential oils

I am going to take it as read that you know how to administer essential oils. If not, please refer to *The Complete Guide to Clinical Aromatherapy and Essential Oils for the Physical Body* where it is explained at length.

I am aware of the possible adulteration issues of solvents, but I still find the healing element of the plant remains and so I am not only drawn to oils which have been extracted by distillation.

Some of the oils I recommend here are hazardous, perhaps because of their strength or for other conditions. I have listed contraindications in each section. Often I use a homeopathic dose, which is 1/15th of a drop. Simply add one drop of essential oil to 14 drops of carrier and then use one drop of the solution.

I would recommend using massage oils during your appointment but also make ranges for them to use at home. Creams, lotions and even evaporator oils will all enhance your treatment effects.

Oils to cleanse the liver, support the adrenals, coax the pituitary

Liver: Rosemary, carrot, eucalyptus

Adrenals : mandarin and camomile

Pituitary: nutmeg, celery seed

Clearly you can use the mentioned acupressure points to help stimulate this further.

Oils to remove toxicity

To recap quickly:

Your best oil to get rid of fertilisers and organic pesticides is oakmoss resin. This oil now has restrictions on it since there were some desensitisation issues in the perfume industry. It can no longer be used in dilutions in excess of 0.1%.

Benzoin, angelica and amber oils are the best oils for removing pharmaceutical debris.

Lemon verbena removes peroxides. (For example, chlorine in sanitary wear).

Positive ions (fluorescent bulbs, V.D.U. emissions) - Cypress

Heavy metals – Citronella

Radiation – Garlic

Oils for Emotions

In the Mind Body Spirit of Clinical Aromatherapy, we looked at Candace Pert's findings about the connections between neuropeptides and the emotions. Here we have a direct link. She identified CRF (Cortisol Releasing Factor) as being the neuropeptides of negative expectations.

So, then, it is these thoughts that release the cortisol causing the problems. We address the problem from the thought upwards.

Negative expectations:

The main areas we can pinpoint these to, are:

Work, relationships, school, money, siblings, exams/driving test.

It's all too much – *Camomile Maroc* – helps to sink under one's problems. *Helichrysm* – Strengthening.

I will fail – *Frankincense* - for confidence, *Coriander*: Fear of doing **something**; orange- Helps a person see what they are truly capable of.

How are we going to pay? *Geranium* – Interface between mental and emotional for finances

He will leave –*Celery Seed:* Helps understanding of domestic situations.

She will reject me – *Jasmine-* Sexuality issues.

Something bad will happen (lose job etc) – *Black Pepper* – Excellent oil for building constructive teams and keeping groups together

People will look at me – *Spearmint*: Counters embarrassment

People will judge me – *Tangerine*: Near as dammit shouts so f****ng what! (I love an oil with attitude!)

The exam questions will be different to my prep – *Rosewood*: focus; (and some Rescue Remedy)

I will screw up! – Oakmoss – brings half remembered truths from the subconscious to allow them to dissipate.

It will happen again: *Amber*- Lifts trauma

He will hurt me (emotions) - Rose

He will hurt me (brutalise) – Camphor (homeopathic dose)

There will be an argument- *Cade*: Calms arguments, *Mimosa*- Familial bonding, *Mandarin* – convivial atmosphere, *Dill*: Relationships with teenagers

She is better at things than me: *Benzoin*- Helps a person to break free of mental fetters

Essential oils for chakra healing
Some oils which vibrate on the chakras are:

Crown

Frankincense, Palma Rosa, Cumin, Sandalwood,

Brow

Aniseed, Camomile Roman, Cardamom, Clary Sage, Hop,

Jasmine, Camomile Maroc, Carrot, Rose Geranium, Tea Tree, Valerian, Rose Otto (Enfleurage),

Throat

Cypress, Dill, Ginger, Bulgarian Lavender, Rose Otto (Distilled) Peppermint, Neroli

Heart

Amber, Basil, Bay, Benzoin, Lavandin, Mandarin, Orange, Spearmint, Rose Maroc, Rose geranium,

Cajuput, Lavender, Peppermint, Neroli

Sacral

Black Pepper, Tonka Bean, Peppermint, Rose Otto (Distilled)

Base or root

Clove

For a more in depth understanding of how the oils will affect the chakras and the etheric bodies of the aura, please see: Jill Bruce's Garden of Eden, as well as her book The Aura. There are dozens more oils for you to choose from there. For a better understanding of which emotions correspond to which organ, please refer to *The Mind Body Spirit of Clinical Aromatherapy.*

Yin /Yang Essential oils

Since all plant medicine is yin, take this to mean Yin – would work as yang, it will raise yin less than yin+. Therefore, oils that are yin – are your best choices, followed by yin neutral. The list is not exhaustive and so I will expect you will add your own. Basically, remember if it is a top note, then you will push yin up. When blending then, of course you will need some top notes but try and weight your blends at the base. Anchor your client down.

Angelica	Yin +
Basil	Yin +
Bay	Yin neutral
Benzoin	Yin -
Bergamot	Yin +
Birch	Yin -
Black Pepper	Yin neutral
Cajuput	Yin neutral
Camomile	Yin neutral
Camphor	Yin -
Caraway	Yin +
Cardamon	Yin neutral
Carrot	Yin +

Cedarwood Atlas	Yin -
Cinnamon	Yin -
Clary Sage	Yin neutral
Clove Bud	Yin -
Coriander	Yin neutral
Cumin	Yin neutral
Cypress	Yin -
Eucalyptus	Yin +
Fennel	Yin neutral
Frankincense	Yin -
Galbanum	Yin -
Geranium	Yin neutral
Ginger	Yin neutral
Grapefruit	Yin +
Hyssop	Yin neutral
Jasmine	Yin -
Juniper	Yin neutral
Lavender	Yin neutral
Lemon	Yin +
Lemon Grass	Yin +
Lemon Verbena	Yin +
Mandarin	Yin +
Marigold	Yin neutral
Marjoram	Yin neutral
Melissa	Yin neutral

Myrrh	Yin -
Myrtle	Yin -
Neroli	Yin -
Nutmeg	Yin +
Oakmoss	Yin -
Orange	Yin +
OregaNo	Yin neutral
Parsley Leaf	Yin neutral
Patchouli	Yin -
Peppermint	Yin neutral
Petitgrain	Yin +
Pimento	Yin neutral
Pine	Yin -
Rose	Yin -
Rosemary	Yin neutral
Rosewood	Yin -
Sage	Yin +
Sandalwood	Yin -
Spearmint	Yin neutral
Tarragon	Yin neutral
Tea Tree	Yin +
Thyme	Yin neutral
Valerian	Yin -
Vertiver	Yin -
Violet Leaf	Yin −

| Ylang Ylang | Yin neutral |

Conclusion

I am flattered and relieved you found your way to this page. It means I have not bored you to death. I love aromatherapy and never cease to be amazed by the wonderful things it can do. This is an exciting time for you to be in the therapy because the world is shifting into your light. We are starting to get noticed. We owe that to people like my Jill and Michael, but also to people like Jeanne Rose, Robert Tisserand, Wanda Sellar, Patricia Davis, Valerie Worwood, Gabriel Mojay, Nicole Perez...the list could go on and on. They believed in their medicine and they went out there and sold it hard.

Now it's your turn. The problem is of course selling doesn't often sit well with gentle souls. Do you have what it takes you find those clients to move your business forward, now you have the tools to heal?

I think yes, in fact I *know* yes and I'll tell you why.

Your own nurturing qualities versus Get out and hunt for your clients

The main reason *any* business fails is a skilled person enters self employment expecting customers will find their way to them because they are good at what they do. They don't actively and deliberately go and hunt out their prey. (Let's be honest it is going in for the kill which is going to put meals on your table now, isn't it?)

In complementary medicine it is worse than many other industries because therapists are quiet, gentle people who do not sit easily with the aggressive persona of classical selling.

I see the successful aromatherapist as a huntress. She is at ease with nature. She is aware at all times of what is happening in her environment. She actually targets where she will find her business and the healing sits behind that. She has carefully structured conversations (not a pitch, you will notice) with the right people at the right time and she walks away with the business. Because her practice is sales lead, she sees more far more clients. She makes more people better and then *healing* success follows in her wake.

It's time to start playing with the big boys...

For the main part aromatherapy is a feminine art. Whilst there are extremely good male therapists, at the pinnacle of the industry Tisserand, Penoel and Mojay to name just a few, statistically the number of women on the practitioners' register far outstrips the number of men.

Herein lays a potential difficulty for essential oil healing as I see it. For the rulers of the sales world are, in the main, men. More saliently the gurus of the internet are predominantly men. So those who are making a killing raking in the revenue from our oils and essential oil information are not potentially healers at all. So then, the *industry* grows but the therapy does not. More to the point, an increasing number of essential oils are being sold to beginners but these interested parties are not finding their ways to practitioners' doors at all. And why? Because the internet is selling essential oils but it is not selling aromatherapy. We need this to change.

So ladies and gentlemen, forget the lavender oil, it's time to wake up and smell the coffee. You simply have to start selling. Don't let that worry you. In *Sales Strategies For Gentle Souls* I'll show you where your customers are, how to target them and even how to maximise your profit margin in the process. It's easy (hard work potentially, but certainly not difficult) and as a woman I can tell you really good quality selling is great fun when you know how.

See you on the other side....

Liz

PS Please don't forget our original deal. Please turn over for details of how to place your review. Review and buy!

Bye!

About the Author

Elizabeth Ashley qualified as an aromatherapist in 1993, and then passed the Advanced Aromatherapy Diploma in 1994. She has been practicing aromatherapy for over 21 years.

In 1999, she fell into a whole new career in the aggressive commercial sector of recruitment consultancy. There she learned her father's second hand car salesman genes had passed along and found she had quite a gift of the gab! More than that, she discovered she could sell...and then some.

In 2008, Elizabeth fell ill during pregnancy with a blood clot in her lungs. The pulmonary embolism prevented her from working and she started to write. Very quickly she gained her first contract as a ghost writer...a recipe book for cheese cakes!

In 2010 She was published professionally for her work on Galbanum oil in the Aromatherapy Thymes, journal of the International Federation of Aromatherapists, and on Tuberose oil by the New Zealand Register of Holistic Therapist.

In 2011 she was seconded, on a consultative basis, to Walsall Independent Treatment Centre, designed to be a rainbow bridge between traditional and complementary medicines. There she became aware of the rumblings of change in healthcare. Her book *Sales Strategies for Gentle Souls* explains the connotations of this.

In 2014 she ranks in the top 50 contract writers on the freelancer marketplace Elance.com. She is the ghost writer of seven number one Amazon best sellers in the natural healing category. She lives in Shropshire with her husband and youngest son, kept company by their cat, the budgie and many shoals of tropical fish! Her elder son and daughter attend university and make her prouder than anything ever could.

Elizabeth Ashley is The Secret Healer. Her books are designed to fill gaps in aromatherapy knowledge and train therapists how to bring their business into the cyber age and make their practices excel.

Other works by the author

Book 1 - The Complete Guide to

Clinical Aromatherapy & Essential Oils for the Physical Body
Essentially...essential oils for beginners, talented novices and intermediate aromatherapists

Let me ask you, why do you want a book on aromatherapy?

Do you want to learn how to care for your family naturally?

Perhaps you have a franchise selling essential oils and want to know more about what they can do?

Maybe you love the delicious scents and want understand how these beautiful things come to heal.

I wonder if you have started to learn and now want to discover how to build on your knowledge.

Whatever you are looking for this book has something for you.

- Details of how to treat over 60 conditions with essential oils
- Profiles of over 100 natural plant essences and their safety data
- Descriptions of 15 carrier oils and their applications not only for massage but also adding to creams and lotions.

- Comprehensive data of how the chemistry of an oil will affect its actions
- In depth insights into how professional aromatherapists blend...including their 13 favourite recipes from their practices.

Including....

- Sensuous aromatherapy blends by a qualified sex therapist
- Two blends for labour by the midwife running an aromatherapy program on an NHS maternity ward
- A blend for depression by a qualified mental health

PLUS....

10 bonus essential oil monographs and a complementary hypnotherapy relaxation download.

Discount vouchers of treatments courses and products by participating therapists.

AND.... for those of you who would like to contribute, there is a chance to make a donation to cancer research too.

This is my gift to you.

FREE - From 30.11.14

Book 2 Essential Oils for Mind Body Spirit

The Holistic Medicine of Clinical Aromatherapy

Healing the skin, easing the tummy ache or getting someone to sleep is easy with essential oils. Anyone can do it. The joy of healing, though, comes from peeling back the layers of the disease, almost like a detective to find out exactly what caused it in the first place.

Consider this book to be lesson 2 in The Secret Healer Series.

You have mastered which oil to use for what and why...this book takes you step by step though the ancient healing mechanisms of the aura, the chakras and meridians but also explores how that ties in with the latest scientific discoveries into how the emotions affect our health. Using Candace Pert's remarkable "Molecules of Emotion" research, The Secret Healer shows you *where* to look for healing links and *why*.

- Uncover how a certain recurrent negative emotion can be the trigger to make you ill?
- Understand internal processes that mean that psychology, neurology and immunology are quintessentially, and inextricably linked.
- Learn how to use essential oils control your emotions and in turn bring about a far greater standard of wellness.

- Discover mindblowing research that shows the emotions we experience are actually the sensations of neuropeptides triggering our organs to do their jobs
- Reflect on the wonder of Chinese medicine and ancient healing being completely accurate in their healing mechanisms for thousands of years...now that science proves it to be so.

Essential Oils for The Mind Body Spirit couples ancient wisdom with cutting edge science. This is the knowledge the drug companies hope you never find out and our doctors pray we all will.

A short write up, for a book that will change your life. I promise you, when you read the latest findings of psychoimmunolgy, you will never waster another day on being angry again.

Book 3 The Essential Oil Liver Cleanse

The Professional Aromatherapist's Liver Detox

We are warned of the threats of heart attacks, strokes and cancer, especially if we are overweight.

What is kept quieter is doctors have established a link between toxicity in the liver and metabolic syndrome, the condition that leads to many of these conditions. What's more non fatty liver disease is known to underlie many other conditions such as eczema, allergies and headaches.

The scandal is just how many of our livers are struggling under the strain of over processed foods, pharmaceutical debris and actually even our own bad tempers!

This book explains:

- The importance of the liver and its functions
- How it becomes dysfunctional and how to interpret warning signposts
- How to cleanse and nourish using not just essential oils, but also vitamins and minerals and diet.
- The strange correlation between how our emotions translate negativity into disease.
- How to implement other therapies such as chiropractic, acupressure and counselling and how to secure fantastic referrals.

This book is best used in tandem with The Professional Stress Solution to benefit from the complementary healing. Use Sales Strategies for Gentle Souls to create a marketing plan to use your new found knowledge to smash your competition out of the water!!!

Book 4 The Professional Stress Solution

Essential Oils and Holistic Health Stress Management Techniques for The Professional Aromatherapist

Stress is pandemic in our society.

Scientists agree it plays a quintessential role in how likely it is we will suffer from chronic and possibly fatal illnesses in the future. Risk factors of metabolic syndrome, diabetes, stroke and heart disease are increased through stress.

The daft thing is....aromatherapy can do amazing things to ease it, and potentially aromatherapists could take a massive workload away from the doctor's surgeries.

- Discover the hormonal changes and peptide triggers that change a person's health and mental state.
- Learn how it affects the liver, adrenals and pituitary gland.
- Uncover the strange phenomenon of Yin disease
- Build a better foundation of care, but also a knowledge base that means you can sell your treatments more effectively.
- Improve your healing skills set
- Supercharge your referrals potential from other complementary therapists and orthodox medicine alike.

Includes free bonus material of

- Chiropractic chart of misalignments and potential organic disturbance
- Chart of the meridians and suggested acupressure points to detox the organs more quickly
- Detailed information about how to improve the patients condition with vitamin and minerals therapy
- In depth dietary advice
- Free hypnotherapy relaxation download

Essential Oils are The Off Switch for stress. The *Professional Stress Solution* is the ON SWITCH for your aromatherapy business.

Book 5 The Aromatherapy Eczema Treatment

Healing Eczema, Itchy Skin Rashes and Atopic Dermatitis with Essential Oils and Holistic Medicine

Most people appreciate that the itching and redness of eczema can be used using essential oils, but what if I told you they were capable of so much more?

Imagine if, as a therapist, you were able to pinpoint the emotions that set off these flares? Can you visualise what it would mean to your patient if you were able to isolate the very protagonist causing the eczema breakout and alleviate their pain completely?

Well now you can.

This book teaches you:

- How to isolate the emotions causing the emotional cycle of pain
- The likely food triggers for your patient and the tools to identify the exact times they will detonate a reaction
- The familial traits and links that lead to atopic eczema
- How these links connect with the liver and in turn how to cleanse the liver toxicity
- Vitamins and minerals to cleanse and nourish the system

The book contains very real that will not only transform the way you treat clients, but will skyrocket your clinic's takings.

I recommend reading this book in tandem with *The Professional Stress Solution* and the *Essential Oil Liver Cleanse* to fully understand the cycles and processes of treatment. Add to it *Sales Strategies for Gentle Souls* and your business will stand on an entirely new footing.

I promise you...nothing else comes even close.

Sales Strategies for Gentle Souls
Targeted Sales Training for Professional Aromatherapists

Wonderful things are happening in complementary therapy. Very gifted people are churning out fantastic research and results. The internet is full of what essential oils can do. But when a gentle soul emerges from their relaxing haze of their aromatherapy class room, how do they harness the buzz of energy around them for their craft?

From 1999-2008 I worked in one of the most aggressive commercial environments there is. My role as a recruitment consultant was 80% cold calling in am extremely saturated sales arena. Despite my own gentle soul, I found ways not only to compete, but to excel.

- Learn how to pinpoint the best customers for your practice
- Cost your treatments to ensure every treatment is profitable for both you and your customer
- Discover how to make every conversation into a potential sale lead without becoming a complete and utter pain in the a*s!
- Uncover the reasons why you are not closing sales so you never have to make the same mistakes again
- Create a growth environment where you plan success and always find yourself stepping into it

If you are working with essential oils, and you want to make a good living for it, then you need to learn to sell. What's more, if you are going to say "selling doesn't work on my customers"....then you have simply been taught to do it wrongly.

My dream is to see aromatherapy at the forefront of medicine. I need an army of gifted healers to achieve that. Consider yourself to be my newest recruit and I am going to drill you till you are the slickest, subtlest and most effective marketeer there is. You have the knowledge to make people better, now let me give you the business prowess to heal even more people than you have ever done before.

The Secret Healer has stress in her sights and she's about to make a killing. Listen carefully...she has much to tell you.

www.thesecrethealer.co.uk

Acknowledgements

There are so many people I want to thank, I feel like Gwyneth Paltrow at the Oscars!

Thanks to my mum and Michael for their generous knowledge.

Here is heartfelt love to my lovely dad. I have so much appreciation for teaching me never to take things at face value.

To Anna for her daily emails, to Mark, Rebecca, Luanne, Angie, Yvette, Ariane, Liz and Oliver for giving me confidence to get this book done. To RobertElsmoreImages, thanks for your patience with my picture changes, again and again.

To Angela and Pauline, I send much gratitude for checking up on me and keeping my feet on the ground. To Pat and Neil for believing in me.

To my children, you are my world and contrary to your opinions, I think this book confirms that I *am*, in fact, cool. To my husband, simply and completely....thanks.

Disclaimer

by SEQ Legal

(1)   Introduction

This disclaimer governs the use of this book. [By using this book, you accept this disclaimer in full. / We will ask you to agree to this disclaimer before you can access the book.]

(2)   Credit

This disclaimer was created using an <u>SEQ Legal</u> template.

(3)   No advice

The book contains information about aromatherapy and the use of essential oils.The information is not advice, and should not be treated as such.

[You must not rely on the information in the book as an alternative to qualified medical advice from a health professional. advice from an appropriately qualified professional. If you have any specific questions about any medical matter you should consult an appropriately qualified professional.]

[If you think you may be suffering from any medical condition you should seek immediate medical attention. You should never delay seeking medical advice, disregard medical advice, or discontinue medical treatment because of information in the book.]

(4) No representations or warranties

To the maximum extent permitted by applicable law and subject to section 6 below, we exclude all representations, warranties, undertakings and guarantees relating to the book.

Without prejudice to the generality of the foregoing paragraph, we do not represent, warrant, undertake or guarantee:

that the information in the book is correct, accurate, complete or non-misleading;

that the use of the guidance in the book will lead to any particular outcome or result; or

in particular, that by using the guidance in the book you will heal disease or work in any way as a cure for illness.

(5) Limitations and exclusions of liability

The limitations and exclusions of liability set out in this section and elsewhere in this disclaimer: are subject to section 6 below; and govern all liabilities arising under the disclaimer or in relation to the book, including liabilities arising in contract, in tort (including negligence) and for breach of statutory duty.

We will not be liable to you in respect of any losses arising out of any event or events beyond our reasonable control.

We will not be liable to you in respect of any business losses, including without limitation loss of or damage to profits, income, revenue, use, production, anticipated savings, business, contracts, commercial opportunities or goodwill.

We will not be liable to you in respect of any loss or corruption of any data, database or software.

We will not be liable to you in respect of any special, indirect or consequential loss or damage.

(6)   Exceptions

Nothing in this disclaimer shall: limit or exclude our liability for death or personal injury resulting from negligence; limit or exclude our liability for fraud or fraudulent misrepresentation; limit any of our liabilities in any way that is not permitted under applicable law; or exclude any of our liabilities that may not be excluded under applicable law.

(7)   Severability

If a section of this disclaimer is determined by any court or other competent authority to be unlawful and/or unenforceable, the other sections of this disclaimer continue in effect.

If any unlawful and/or unenforceable section would be lawful or enforceable if part of it were deleted, that part will be deemed to be deleted, and the rest of the section will continue in effect.

(8)   Law and jurisdiction

This disclaimer will be governed by and construed in accordance with English law, and any disputes relating to this disclaimer will be subject to the exclusive jurisdiction of the courts of England and Wales.

(9)   Our details

In this disclaimer, "we" means (and "us" and "our" refer to) The Secret Healer / buildyourownreality.com, a partnership established under English law having its principal place of business at 4, SY8 1LQ.

Bibliography

Works Cited

Adolphs R1, T. D. (1999 Sep). Recognition of facial emotion in nine individuals with bilateral amygdala damage. *Neuropsychologia.* , 37(10):1111-7.

Bergland, C. (2013, January 22). *Why the stress hormone is public enemy number 1.* Retrieved June 10, 2014, from Psychology   Today: http://www.psychologytoday.com/blog/the-athletes-way/201301/cortisol-why-the-stress-hormone-is-public-enemy-no-1

Bostock, S., & Steptoe, A. (Apr 2013;). Influences of early shift work on the diurnal cortisol rhythm, mood and sleep: Within-subject variation in male airline pilots. *Psychoneuroendocrinology.* , 38(4): 533–541.

Brosnan, M. J.-C.-N. (2009). Absence of a normal Cortisol Awakening Response (CAR) in adolescent males with Asperger Syndrome (AS). . *Psychoneuroendocrinology, 34 (7),* , pp. 1095-1100.

Bruce, J. (1993). How to Treat Stress. *Diploma of Aromatherapy* .

Bruce, J. (2014). *The Aura.* Ludlow: Buildyourownreality.com.

Bruce, J. (1995). *The Garden of Eden*. Walsall: Magdelena Press.

Bruce, J. (n.d.). Vitamins and Minerals. *Advanced Diploma of Aromatherapy* . Aromatherapy, Jill Bruce School of.

Bryant R.A., F. K.-S. (67(12), 1217-1219. doi:10.1016/j.biopsych.2010.03.016). Preliminary Evidence of the Short Allele of the Serotonin Transporter Gene Predicting Poor Response to Cognitive Behavior Therapy in Posttraumatic Stress Disorder. *Biological Psychiatry,* .

Cahill, L., Haier, R., White, N., Fallon, J., Kilpatrick, L., Lawrence, C., et al. (2001). Sex-Related Difference in Amygdala Activity during Emotionally Influenced Memory Storage. *Neurobiology of Learning and Memory* , 75 (1): 1–9.

Cook, M. (1994). Medical Dowsing Course.

Damasio, A. (1999). *The Feeling of What Happens: Body, Emotion and the Making of Consciousness*. London: Heinemann .

Department of Biological Sciences, S. U.-5. (2001, Oct 23). Depression, antidepressants, and the shrinking hippocampus. *Proc Natl Acad Sci U S A.* , pp. 98(22): 12320–12322.

E. Sherwood Brown, P. M. (Feb 2001;). Mood and Cognitive Changes During Systemic Corticosteroid Therapy. *Prim Care Companion J Clin Psychiatry.* , 3(1): 17–21.

Hamann, S. (2005). Sex Differences in the Responses of the Human Amygdala. *Neuroscience update* , 11 (4): 288.

http://www.stress.org/stress-effects/. (1999). *50 Common Signs of Stress*. Retrieved June 10, 2014, from The American Institute of Stress: http://www.stress.org/stress-effects/

Hudson, G. (n.d.). Retrieved from http://www.guyhudson.co.uk.

Johansen, P.-Ø., & Technology, T. K. (Jan 2010). Ecstasy For Treatment Of Traumatic Anxiety. *Psychopharmacology*.

K. GUGGENHEIM, S. H. (1953). *The effects of antibiotics on the metabolism of certain B vitamins*. Retrieved from http://jn.nutrition.org/content/50/2/245.full.pdf

Kim, P. A., & School, M. H. (2006). Anxiogenic-Like Effect of Chronic Corticosterone in the Light–Dark Emergence Task in Mice. *Behavioural Neuroscience* , Vol. 120, No. 2, 249 –256.

M.D., D. L. (n.d.). Retrieved from http://www.drlwilson.com/.

McEwen BS1, S. E. (1993 , Sep 27). Stress and the individual. Mechanisms leading to disease. *Arch Intern Med.* , pp. 153(18):2093-101.

Melissa A. Bright1, *. D. (2011). Do infants show an awakening cortisol response? *Dev. Psychobiol.* , 54: 736–743. doi: 10.1002/dev.20617.

Nigel F Huddleston BSc, P. C. (n.d.). *http://synthesislearning.com/article/brwav.htm.* Retrieved from synthesislearning.com: http://synthesislearning.com/article/brwav.htm

Sonino N1, F. G. (1998 Nov-Dec;). Clinical correlates of major depression in Cushing's disease. *Psychopathology.* , 31(6):302-6.

Swaab*, D. F. (2008). Sexual orientation and its basis in brain structure and function. *Proc Natl Acad Sci U S A* , 105(30): 10273–10274.

Tamashiro KL1, S. R. (2011 Sep;14(5):468-74. doi: 10.3109/10253890.2011.606341.). *Chronic stress, metabolism, and metabolic syndrome.* Baltimore, MD 21205, USA: Department of Psychiatry & Behavioral Sciences, Johns Hopkins University School of Medicine, .

West, N. (n.d.). *Emotions and the organs.* Retrieved from My Holistic Healing.com: My-Holisti-Healing.com

www.ingramcontent.com/pod-product-compliance
Lightning Source LLC
Chambersburg PA
CBHW070707290526
45790CB00001B/480